ESTROGENS
AND
CANCER

ESTROGENS
AND
CANCER

Edited by

Steven G. Silverberg, M.D.
Francis J. Major, M.D.

Colorado Regional Cancer Center and
University of Colorado School of Medicine
Denver

A WILEY MEDICAL PUBLICATION
JOHN WILEY & SONS
New York / Chichester / Brisbane / Toronto

Library of Congress Cataloging in Publication Data:

Main entry under title:

Estrogens and cancer.

  (A Wiley medical publication)
  Based on a symposium sponsored by the Colorado
Regional Cancer Center and the University of Colorado
Medical Center.
    1. Endometrium—Cancer—Etiology—Congresses.
2. Estrogen—Therapeutic use—Side effects—Congresses.
3. Breast—Cancer—Etiology—Congresses. 4. Oral contraceptives—
Side effects—Congresses. 5. Hormone receptors—
Congresses. I. Silverberg, S. G. II. Major, Francis J.
III. Colorado Regional Cancer Center. [DNLM:
1. Estrogens—Adverse effects. 2. Neoplasms—Etiology.
WP522 E81]
RC280.U8E87   616.9'94'071   78-17275
ISBN 0-471-04172-6

Printed in the United States of America

10 9 8 7 6 5 4 3 2 1

Contributors

George Betz, M.D., Ph.D., Department of Obstetrics and Gynecology, University of Colorado School of Medicine, Denver, Colorado 80262

Paul A. Bloustein, M.D., Department of Laboratory Medicine, Wesley Medical Center, Wichita, Kansas 67202

Clarence E. Ehrlich, M.D., Department of Obstetrics and Gynecology, University of Indiana School of Medicine, Indianapolis, Indiana 46202

Lawrence H. Einhorn, M.D., Department of Medicine, Section of Oncology, Indiana University Medical Center, Indianapolis, Indiana 46202

Jack A. Faraci, M.D., Department of Obstetrics and Gynecology, University of Colorado School of Medicine, Denver, Colorado 80262

Robert E. Fechner, M.D., Department of Pathology, The University of Virginia School of Medicine, Charlottesville, Virginia 22903

Veeba Gerkins, M.P.H., Department of Pathology, University of Southern California, School of Medicine, Los Angeles, California 90033

Annlia Hill, Ph.D., Department of Community Medicine, University of Southern California, School of Medicine, Los Angeles, California 90033

Thomas Mack, M.D., Department of Community Medicine, University of Southern California, School of Medicine, Los Angeles, California 90033

Francis J. Major, M.D., Department of Obstetrics and Gynecology, Denver General Hospital and University of Colorado School of Medicine, Denver, Colorado 80202

Edgar L. Makowski, M.D., Department of Obstetrics and Gynecology, University of Colorado School of Medicine, Denver, Colorado 80262

Alexander Miller, M.D., Department of Pathology, Rush Medical School, Chicago, Illinois 60612

John McLean Morris, M.D., Department of Obstetrics and Gynecology, Yale University School of Medicine, New Haven, Connecticut 06516

Dennis Mullen, M.D., Department of Pathology, University of Colorado School of Medicine, Denver, Colorado 80262

Jaime Prat, M.D., Department of Pathology, Massachusetts General Hospital, Boston, Massachusetts 02114

Stanley Robboy, M.D., Department of Pathology, Massachusetts General Hospital, Boston, Massachusetts 02114

Ronald Ross, M.D., Department of Pathology, University of Southern California, School of Medicine, Los Angeles, California 90033

Steven G. Silverberg, M.D., Colorado Regional Cancer Center and Department of Pathology, University of Colorado School of Medicine, Denver, Colorado 80262

Sheldon C. Sommers, M.D., Department of Pathology, Lenox Hill Hospital, New York, New York 10021

Bruce V. Stadel, M.D., M.P.H., National Institute of Child Health and Human Development, National Institutes of Health, Bethesda, Maryland 20014

Noel S. Weiss, M.D., Department of Epidemiology, University of Washington and Fred Hutchinson Cancer Research Center, Seattle, Washington 98195

William R. Welch, M.D., Department of Pathology, Massachusetts General Hospital, Boston, Massachusetts 02114

Peter C. M. Young, Ph.D., Department of Obstetrics and Gynecology, Indiana University Medical Center, Indianapolis, Indiana 46202

Preface

In the past few years, the subject of the multifaceted relationships between exogenous estrogen administration and the development of human tumors has become one of major practical as well as theoretical interest and importance. The recent demonstration of an almost epidemic increase in the incidence of endometrial carcinoma in this country has served to focus the attention of numerous investigators on the stimulation of the development of this tumor by endogenous and exogenous estrogenic hormones. Similarly, investigators have questioned the relationship of estrogens to other tumors and tumor-like conditions of the breast, cervix, vagina, and liver. The agents involved have included conjugated estrogens administered to postmenopausal women, estrogen-progesterone combinations administered as oral contraceptives, and diethylstilbestrol (DES) and related compounds administered during pregnancy.

Because large volumes of often conflicting data have been presented on these subjects in a very short time, and because serious questions still exist concerning not only the interpretation of these data but their translation into alternative courses of action, the Colorado Regional Cancer Center and the University of Colorado Medical Center co-sponsored an invitational symposium, "Estrogens and Cancer," in Denver on September 10, 1977. The presentations at this symposium form the substance of this book.

The goal of this book is to bring together epidemiologic, clinical, and pathologic data on the relationships between estrogens and naturally occurring human neoplasms, and to provide in a single source a compendium of current knowledge and future research directions in a variety of estrogenic compounds and human tumors. Specific objectives include the presentation of both sides of the estrogen-endometrial cancer controversy; ongoing investigations of the relation of postmenopausal estrogens, oral contraceptives, and in utero exposure to DES to human tumors and tumor-like conditions of various sites; and potential therapeutic uses of information relating to estrogen responsiveness of some tumors through the mechanism of the determination of receptor activity.

This volume begins with a general consideration of estrogen metabolism and the pathophysiology of menopause by Dr. Betz and of the treatment of menopausal signs and symptoms by Dr. Morris. The relationship between postmenopausal estrogen administration and endometrial cancer is discussed from different points of view by Drs. Weiss, Miller, and Sommers, while the current status of the relation of postmenopausal estrogen administration to breast cancer is presented by Dr. Ross. These presentations are followed by a discussion of the risk/benefit ratios of postmenopausal estrogen administration. The status of oral contraceptives with relation to endometrial cancer, cervical and mammary cancers, and liver tumors is examined by Drs. Silverberg, Stadel, and Bloustein, respectively. Dr. Fechner presents an update of the pathology of oral contraceptive-related lesions. Another discussion follows on the relationship between contraception and cancer. Finally, Dr. Robboy discusses the current status of the relationship of in utero DES exposure and cervicovaginal cancer and other abnormalities, and Dr. Ehrlich gives an update on estrogen and progesterone receptors and cancer treatment.

As editors, we wish to thank the above-mentioned authors and their colleagues for their excellent contributions and their cooperation in helping us expedite the book's timely publication. We also thank our colleagues at the Colorado Regional Cancer Center and the University of Colorado Medical Center for their assistance with the many difficult organizational aspects of publishing a book such as this in the shortest possible time. We single out for particular praise and thanks Miss Virginia Brookhouser, who handled the administrative and organizational component of the symposium, and Mrs. Lavonne King, who typed the major portion of the manuscript. We also sincerely appreciate the cooperation of John Wiley & Sons, particularly of Miss Ruth Wreschner of their editorial staff. The cooperation and assistance of these and many other people has been invaluable to us in the text's preparation.

Steven G. Silverberg, M.D.
Francis J. Major, M.D.

Contents

Estrogen Metabolism and Pathophysiology of Menopause

George Betz, M.D., Ph.D.

The consequences of the menopausal syndrome are manifold. Although many women undergo this biologic transition without overwhelming difficulty, estrogen deprivation in conjunction with the effects of aging may be devastating to some individuals. Because of the large population segment in this female age group, menopause deserves the attention afforded any public health problem. Fortunately for the impetus of research in this area, the profound endocrine and metabolic alterations attendant to ovarian failure have fascinated investigators. This discussion will attempt to summarize recent advances in our understanding of menopausal biology, including alterations of sex steroid biochemistry and the metabolic consequences of estrogen deprivation.

Age at the cessation of ovarian function has been reported to have increased over the past century, with the mean age changing from 45 to 50. Because of differences in reporting this kind of data between the present time and a century ago, these comparisons may not be reliable (1). The mean age of menopause (50 years) is currently the same in all industrialized nations studied, and the standard deviation of 3.8 years reported from The Netherlands is a representative value (2). The lower values for mean age of menopause, which have been observed currently in undeveloped countries, are probably a consequence of limited nutrition (3). The significance of other factors that might affect the age of menopause has not been established, with the possible exception of altitude (4). Thus, there appears to be no correlation among mean age of menopause and parity, age at menarche, body weight, or intercurrent disease states. The proportion of the population who have reached menopause is reported to be greater than 30% in England (5). Dewhurst has estimated that one fourth of these patients will seek medical help for problems related to menopause (6). To reiterate a previous statement concerning menopause, we are dealing with a major public health problem.

ETIOLOGY OF MENOPAUSE

Causative factors in the onset of the menopausal syndrome have not been clarified. Animal models of menopause require that primates be studied, since lower animals do not shed their endometrium. These observations have not been extensively recorded, and menopause is not well documented in primates other than humans partly because of their shorter life-span. A decline in fertility has been noted in laboratory animals, such as rats, and this decline is primarily manifested by decreases in litter size and in the frequency of gestation. In contrast to human ovaries at menopause, in which a drastic decline in the number of follicles occurs, the morphology of rat ovaries is not extensively altered (7). The decrease in fecundity of rodents appears to be due to uterine changes rather than to the ovarian failure that occurs in human menopause. Some of the events that lead to menopause have been recorded, and it is well documented in human females that cycle length decreases by 2–4 days in the final reproductive years (8, 9). In the final year, anovulation and gross menstrual irregularity are the rule. It was determined that the observed abbreviation of ovulatory cycles was due to a decreased length of the preovulatory phase of the cycle (9), whereas corpus luteum function continued for the usual duration of 14 days. Progesterone and luteinizing hormone (LH) were measured at the same levels as in younger women, but follicle-stimulating hormone (FSH) was increased markedly during the late proliferative phase of perimenopausal women. At the same time, estradiol levels were below normal. This apparent dissociation in the control of LH and FSH opens speculation concerning the factors that modulate the levels of these hormones. It is possible that follicles produce a substance analogous to testicular "inhibin," a hypothetical substance that appears to suppress FSH levels in men. Thus, inhibin may be a major factor in control of FSH, while LH is controlled by estrogen. The finding of a high FSH/LH ratio also corroborates an earlier finding that FSH is inversely related to the number of ovarian follicles, while LH is not as reliable an indicator of follicular status (10). When cycles finally become anovulatory, estradiol increases after the LH surge, but there is no resultant increase in progesterone.

Although decreased numbers of follicles are found in the perimenopausal ovary, significant numbers of follicles persist after cessation of menses (11). Therefore, the cessation of estrogen production in the physiologic menopause does not occur by exactly the same mechanism as in Turner's syndrome, in which no follicles are present. Nevertheless, the report by Fang et al. (12) may be of importance in understanding ovarian failure. These investigators found a spontaneous increase in sex chromosome monosomy with advancing age (third decade compared to seventh decade) in gonadal tissue. Somatic tissues did not demonstrate this change. Unfortunately, the proportion of XO cells at age 70 is only 3%. To invoke this loss of chromosomal material as a cause of ovarian failure will require other information.

Another interesting speculation is that menopausal follicles lose their receptors to LH or FSH or become desensitized to gonadotropins. The techniques required to solve this problem are currently under development but have not been applied to menopausal biology.

STEROIDS IN MENOPAUSE

Steroid hormone production undergoes marked changes during menopause. The most striking alteration is, of course, the decline in estrogen synthesis. This change has recently been studied by measurement of estrogen production rates. This technique estimates the quantity of a hormone that leaves the circulation over a given time period (which should nearly equal the quantity that enters the blood). It is necessary to determine the blood clearance rate, which is accomplished by injecting the radiolabeled hormone of interest intravenously and then determining its disappearance rate by sampling at subsequent intervals. The clearance rate, expressed as milliliters of blood per 24 hr, is multiplied by the blood concentration of the hormone (micrograms/milliliter) to yield a production rate in micrograms per 24 hr. Although this calculation gives an estimate of daily synthesis, this method gives no information about the source of the steroid, as is determined by secretion rates where the tissue of origin is known. These techniques may be utilized, however, to estimate the percentage conversion of one steroid to another in the peripheral circulation, and a quantitative calculation may be made of the amount of hormone derived from circulating precursors. Hormone synthesis in nonendocrine tissue is described as "extraglandular." In determining production rates, it was found that the blood concentration of two of the estrogens decreased from premenopausal levels of about 100 pg/ml to 13 and 30 pg/ml (13) for estradiol and estrone, respectively. Clearance rates for each estrogen were decreased by 20% (estradiol, 790 liters/24 hr/m² to 580 liters/24 hr/m²) (14). Production rates of estradiol in the normal menstrual cycle were found to fluctuate from 80 to 500 μg/day, and estrone production varied from 90 to 300 μg/day, with the highest production occurring prior to ovulation. From the above measurements, it was found that after menopause, estradiol production declines to 12 μg/day and estrone to 45 μg/day (13, 14). As may be noted, estrone is now more significant, quantitatively, than estradiol, which was the predominant estrogen in reproductive years. The reduced clearance rates observed for both estrogens are probably due to a mass action effect of decreased substrate for metabolic processes. There appears to be no quantitative difference in estrogen decline or ultimate levels attained whether ovarian failure occurs as a result of surgery, radiation, or menopause. The decrease of estradiol always exceeds that of estrone (13).

Androgen production after ovarian failure also is changed. The mean concentration of androstenedione declines by one half, while testosterone decreases very little after physiologic menopause (15). Production rates of testosterone in one report were almost unchanged from pre- to postmenopause (16), while the production rate of androstenedione was reduced from 3 to 1.5 mg/day (17). The concentrations of several other steroids are also decreased over 50%, including dehydroepiandrosterone and its ester sulfate (18). This finding is surprising because these steroids are predominately adrenal in origin in premenopausal women. The ²¹C compounds 17-hydroxypregnenolone and 17-hydroxyprogesterone were also lower after menopause (18, 19).

In summary, menopause is associated with a profound decrement in estradiol, but the decrease in estrone is much less marked. Androstenedione concentration and production decrease to 50%, but testosterone decreases only slightly. De-hydroepiandrosterone and its sulfate, 17-hydroxyprogesterone, and 17-hydroxypregnenolone also decrease after menopause.

Steroid Hormone Source

The source of steroid hormones in the postmenopausal female has attracted much research interest. It was previously thought that although the post-menopausal ovary had little function, some reserve for estrogen production persisted to a variable degree in individual patients. This tissue was thought to be the site of estrone production, which was equal to that of the early follicular phase of premenopausal females (20).

The adrenal gland has also been suspect as a de novo source of estrogens, but direct catheterization revealed that the quantities of phenolic steroids in the adrenal vein effluent are very low (21). In contrast, suppression of adrenal activity by administration of dexamethasone to postmenopausal women produced a 75% decrease in estrone concentration but no significant change in estradiol (22). Similarly, ACTH administration to oophorectomized, post-menopausal females causes a doubling of estrogen excretion (23).

To further diminish the role of the postmenopausal ovary in estradiol synthesis, no change in the production rate of this steroid was noted following ovariectomy in postmenopausal women (24). It was also demonstrated that the post-menopausal ovary in vitro retained no capacity for estrogen synthesis when incubated with radioactive precursors (25). In addition, measurement of differences in estrone and estradiol in peripheral blood and ovarian venous effluent indicated that the role of the postmenopausal ovary in the production of these estrogens was negligible (26).

The postmenopausal ovary has, however, been shown to retain some steroidogenic activity. In vitro conversion of pregnenolone to ^{19}C compounds has been demonstrated in postmenopausal ovarian tissue (25). There is also a marked difference in the concentration of the steroids testosterone and androstenedione in ovarian and peripheral venous blood of postmenopausal women, and a significant correlation exists between testosterone (but not androstenedione) concentrations from these sources (26). These authors suggest that testosterone secretion may be higher after menopause as a result of elevated gonadotropin levels, and other investigators have also arrived at this conclusion (27). This increase in testosterone may explain the hirsutism and other signs of defeminization that sometimes appear after menopause. To corroborate the role of gonadotropin in postmenopausal testosterone synthesis, it has been shown that estrogen administration decreases the blood concentration of this androgen (15). Quantitative estimates, arrived at from studies conducted before and after ovariectomy, indicated that the postmenopausal ovary contributes greater than 50% of the total testosterone production, but only 20% of the androstenedione came from this tissue (15, 19). In an extensive study, Vermeulen (28), using differential suppression and stimulation (dexamethasone, ACTH, human chorionic gonadotropin) demonstrated that in the postmenopausal female, progesterone and 17-hydroxyprogesterone are adrenal in origin and that dehydroepiandrosterone and its ester sulfate are secreted mostly by the adrenal. Testosterone, dihydrotestosterone, and androstenedione are both ovarian and adrenal in origin. All of the above steroids demonstrated a diurnal variation, which is consistent with the concept of adrenal participation in synthesis.

As previously noted, the decrement in dehydroepiandrosterone ester sulfate is much in excess of that expected, because most (90%) of this steroid is adrenal in origin. Abraham and Maroulis (29) reported that estrogen apparently has an affect on adrenal steroidogenesis, since dehydroepiandrosterone and its ester sulfate are both restored to near normal concentrations by estrogen treatment. The mechanism of this effect of estrogen is not clear.

Thus, the roles of the postmenopausal ovary and adrenal gland in androgen production seem to be established. It is also unlikely that the postmenopausal ovary plays any role in estrogen secretion. The role of the adrenal gland in postmenopausal estrogen secretion was not immediately apparent, as direct sampling of adrenal effluent yields no estrogenic substances. It was clear, however, that manipulation of adrenal activity by suppression or stimulation leads to marked changes in the concentration of estrone. These findings led to the conclusion that the adrenal gland synthesizes a precursor of estrone and that because of the structural similarities between the steroids, the most likely precursor was androstenedione.

Estrone Production

Estrone production in the postmenopausal woman and the factors that affect this process have been the objects of much study. The possibility that androgens are the precursors of estrone has been recognized since the finding that administration of testosterone to men increased estrogen excretion (30). The possibility that androgen is a substrate for an aromatase activity, not located in steroid-synthesizing tissue, was realized 20 years later (31). This experiment involved administration of testosterone to oophorectomized, adrenalectomized females and demonstrated a resultant increase in estrogen excretion.

The role of androstenedione as a substrate for extraglandular aromatization, in contrast to the role of testosterone, becomes apparent when the quantities of each steroid are considered. In the postmenopausal female, the production rate of testosterone is 350 μg/day (16). Since only 0.12% conversion to estradiol occurs (32), this androgen could account for only a few micrograms of estrogen production. Androstenedione production, at 1500 μg/day, with a conversion of 1.3%, is a more significant source of estrogen. This quantity of estrone still is only 20 μg/day and is less than that found in the early proliferative phase of the menstrual cycle. This value is also less than the reported postmenopausal production rate of 40–50 μg/day (13, 14). It was then reported by Siiteri and MacDonald (20) that in contrast to premenopausal women, in whom the extent of conversion of androstenedione to estrone is 1.3%, the conversion in post-menopausal women is more than doubled. If the total estrone production is determined by the standard isotope dilution method and the result compared to the amount of estrone synthesized from androstenedione conversion, the results are nearly identical. Thus, the entire source of estrone in the postmenopausal female is from extraglandular conversion of androstenedione (20).

These observations led to further interesting postulates by the above authors (20). In a study of postmenopausal patients with a history of abnormal bleeding, increased estrone production was found. This abnormal estrone synthesis might have been due to increased quantity of precursor or to an increase in the conversion fraction. Instead of the usual 2–3% conversion, these patients demonstrated conversion of up to 9%. The most obvious factor in common about these patients was that their mean body weight was 100 lb above normal. A subsequent study that involved more patients showed a strong correlation between body weight and percentage conversion of androstenedione to estrone. A logical explanation of this increase in conversion is that adipose tissue has an active aromatizing system. At least two in vitro experiments have demonstrated such conversion in fat tissue (33, 34), although activities are low.

Further support for the role of obesity in abnormal estrone synthesis comes from the studies by Judd et al. (35). In these experiments, blood estrone and estradiol concentrations were found to correlate significantly with body weight and excess weight in these obese patients. As anticipated, ovariectomy did not alter estrogen concentration nor was there a correlation among height, age, or years after the menopause. A weight-matched group of patients was studied with and without endometrial carcinoma. No difference in estrogen concentration was found between these two groups.

An extensive study undertaken to further clarify the significance of the conversion percentage (androstenedione to estrone) was reported by Rizkallah et al. (36). They determined conversion fractions by simultaneous injection of $[^{14}C]$-androstenedione (A) and $[^3H]$estrone (E_1), as described by Siiteri and MacDonald (20). Urine was collected for 5 days. Estrone was isolated and recrystallized until constant isotopic ratios were attained. The conversion fraction equals

$$\frac{R^I E_1 - {}^3H}{R^I A - {}^{14}C} \div \frac{{}^3H}{{}^{14}C} E_1,$$

where R^I is the amount of radioactivity infused. Tritiated estrone serves as an internal standard, and this calculation represents the amount of androstenedione aromatized at the tissue site rather than reflecting androstenedione excreted as a urinary metabolite of estrone. Rizkallah et al. point out that the mathematical model on which these calculations of conversions are based (37) is only valid under certain conditions. It is requisite that both isotopic forms of estrone undergo the same metabolic fate as the endogenous hormone. This condition might not be met because of metabolism of the tracers prior to mixing. Because of the numerous tissues that are known to effect aromatization, variations in conversion ratio would add complex factors to the above equation. Any product of androstenedione aromatization other than estrone would also result in miscalculation. Further considerations include metabolic isotope effects and variable release rates of estrone from extravascular compartments. The conclusion was reached that conversion fractions calculated by the above equation can be little better than rough approximations of the true value. Nevertheless, these authors found a strong correlation between excess weight (above ideal weight) or the height/weight ratio and conversion fraction. They also found an increase in conversion fractions after menopause. The conversion fraction also correlated strongly with the estrone production rate determined by isotopic dilution in patients who had abnormal endometrium (carcinoma, hyperplasia) but not in postmenopausal women with normal endometrium. The reason for this difference is not clear. Thus, although the exact meaning of the conversion fraction is unknown, the method of calculation yields a value with some significance.

In contrast to the above paper, which is in partial agreement with the work of Siiteri and MacDonald, the work of Marshall et al. (38) suggests that the conversion fraction is of limited consequence. These investigators find no correlation between conversion rate and body weight. Instead, they present evidence to show that the plasma concentration of androstenedione is the critical factor in determining estrone concentration. A comparison of estrone concentrations in four groups of patients (perimenopausal, postmenopausal, postovariectomy, posthysterectomy) was undertaken. The mean value of estrone in the perimenopausal group was about twice that of the other groups. The same finding occurred when androstenedione was measured. Correlation of the two steroid concentrations is found in each of the above groups, suggesting that the cause of elevated estrone was a high level of androstenedione. In an abstract, Siiteri and coworkers (39) state that they observed elevated androstenedione production rates in patients with endometrial cancer.

Although many uncertainties exist, the source and significance of postmenopausal estrone production are being elucidated. Several studies cited herein show a relation between estrone synthesis and either endometrial cancer, hyperplasia, or such factors as obesity, which are related to cancer. It is also true that several studies demonstrate no correlation between steroid metabolism and cancer and that many patients with endometrial cancer are of normal weight. Siiteri et al. (40) have postulated that long-term exposure to estrone in the virtual absence of other estrogens may be a critical factor in the genesis of estrogen-related tumors.

METABOLIC CONSEQUENCES OF THE MENOPAUSE

The metabolic and tropic alterations that occur after menopause have not been fully delineated. It is known that estrogen plays a role in the most striking immediate symptom of menopause, the hot flash. Known target tissue, such as vaginal mucosa, undergoes involution in the absence of estrogen. These problems are easily managed, if necessary, by estrogen administration. Much evidence has also accumulated that postmenopausal osteoporosis develops as a result of estrogen deprivation. The role of the menopause in coronary artery disease in women is much less clear, and understanding of the effects of estrogen on such tissues as skin also requires more investigation. The lack of estrogen as a cause of perimenopausal psychiatric problems is particularly difficult to unravel. Certainly, hot flashes and atropic vaginitis are a further threat to femininity that is already threatened by cessation of menses. Estrogen therapy is not adequate treatment for a menopausal involutional psychosis, but such treatment may be helpful as adjunctive therapy. Because of a paucity of factual information about other facets of menopause, this discussion will be limited to the available information concerning osteoporosis and coronary artery disease.

Osteoporosis

The presence of osteoporosis has been a major rationale for the administration of estrogen to postmenopausal women. Up to 25% of women over age 60 may suffer fractures from this disorder. The original classic publication relating these two syndromes was published in 1941 by Albright et al. and promoted the theory that the absence of estrogen's anabolic activity resulted in a decrease in osteoid. Absence of osteoid, the protein matrix for mineralization, led to a decrease in bone strength (42). Since that time, it has been recognized that several factors, such as diet and activity, play a role in the development of osteoporosis. There does appear to be a definite association of bone loss with menopause (43), and this change is more nearly related to the duration of estrogen deprivation than to age (44). The original concept of estrogen's relationship to bone tissue is much more complex, however, than the effect of a positive nitrogen balance induced by the hormone. Over the past decade, it has been realized that estrogen, instead of promoting bone mineralization, acts to prevent bone resorption (45) and thus is an antagonist of parathyroid hormone, among other factors that cause bone turnover. It is therefore not surprising that estrogen has never been reported to be effective in promoting remineralization of osteoporotic bone.

In contrast, several studies cited in a recent review by Heaney (46) demonstrate that postmenopausal bone loss can be prevented by estrogen in daily doses as low as 23 μg of mestranol. The clinical significance of these findings is clouded by the fact that no study has spanned the latent period from menopause to the onset of osteoporotic fractures, which may be 15 years in duration. The only study that purports to demonstrate fracture protection is based on a difference in height loss between treated and untreated groups (47).

In summary, there is good evidence that estrogen therapy will prevent the bone loss associated with menopause. There is only fragmentary data to indicate that the effects of estrogen will be clinically significant in preventing fractures. Since postmenopausal osteoporosis affects only one of five women, it would be helpful if a prediction could be made as to which patients should be treated. Unfortunately, no such predictions can be made concerning women at risk for fracture.

Cardiovascular Disease

Prevention of cardiovascular disease has also been the object of postmenopausal estrogen replacement. The employment of this therapy was based on the apparent fact that women seem to be protected from coronary artery disease until menopause (48). It was also noted that estrogen reversed serum lipid profiles associated with coronary artery disease (49). Another early study that supports this application of estrogens demonstrated inhibition, and even disappearance, of coronary atheromata in estrogen-treated chicks (50). These observations led to the treatment with estrogen of groups of men who had had a single myocardial infarction. Instead of the anticipated absence of recurrence, a sevenfold increase in cardiovascular problems occurred. This result occurred in the first 2 months of treatment and predominated in those who received 10 mg of Premarin (51). After reducing the dosage, a decrease in overall mortality was observed after 5 years of treatment. In contrast, a study that utilized ethynylestradiol in a similar group of men showed a higher mortality in the estrogen-treated group (52). To further confuse the role of estrogen in vascular disease, a recent report relates oral contraceptives to an increased risk of myocardial infarction in older women (53).

Some reasons for this confusion are now apparent. Epidemiologic data from the Framingham Study have recently again been reported (54). No sharp increase in coronary artery disease was observed at menopause, and women are still at much lower risk than are men until age 75. The only effect of menopause was noted in young women (age 40–44). In this group, postmenopausal women (natural or surgical menopause) were at much greater risk than were women with intact ovarian function. Their risk still did not approach that of men. Currently, blood triglyceride levels are considered a major risk factor in coronary artery disease. Estrogen has been shown to increase blood concentrations of these lipids (55). Studies of atheroma inhibition in chicks could not be duplicated in other species. Retrospective studies of heart disease in women undergoing oophorectomy have been reviewed (49), and the results do not show a clear-cut difference between women who had surgery and controls.

The case for ovarian failure as a cause of coronary atherosclerosis is far from convincing. The only well-controlled data seem to be from the Framingham Study, which shows that younger women may be at risk because of ovarian failure.

CONCLUSIONS

The factors that lead to physiologic ovarian failure are almost completely unknown. Some information is available concerning the hormonal events that immediately precede menopause. The changes that occur in steroid metabolism after menopause have been well studied, and it is known that the major estrogen, estrone, is derived from conversion of androgens. There are data to link this conversion fraction to body weight and thus to endometrial cancer. The major metabolic effect of estrogen deprivation that has been established is the effect of the hormone on bone. Estrogen stabilizes bone and thus prevents resorption but does not promote calcification. An effect of estrogen in preventing coronary artery disease has only minimal scientific basis.

REFERENCES

1. Frommer DJ: Brit Med J **2:**349, 1964.
2. Jaszmann LJB: in *The Management of the Menopause and Post-Menopausal Years*, Campbell S (ed.), London, MTP Press, 1976, p. 11.
3. Scragg RFR: Annual Symposium of the New Guinea Medical Society, 1973.

4. Cruz-Coke R: Meeting of Investigators on Population Biology of Altitude, Washington, DC.
5. Gray RH: in *The Menopause*, Beard RJ (ed.), Baltimore, University Park Press, 1976, p. 25.
6. Dewhurst J: in *The Management of the Menopause and Post-Menopausal Years*, Campbell S (ed.), London, MTP Press, 1976, p. 25.
7. Thorneycroft IH, Soderwall AL: Anat Rec **165**:343, 1969.
8. Treloar AE, Boynton RE, Benn BG, et al: Int J Fertil **12**:77, 1967.
9. Sherman BM, West JH, Korenman SG: J Clin Endocrinol Metab **42**:629, 1976.
10. Goldenberg RL, Grodin JM, Rodbard D, et al: Amer J Obstet Gynecol **116**:1003, 1973.
11. Block E: Acta Anat **14**:108, 1952.
12. Fang JS, Jagiello G, Ducayen M, et al: Obstet Gynecol **45**:455, 1975.
13. Mikhail G: Amer J Obstet Gynecol **116**:1069, 1973.
14. Longcope C: Amer J Obstet Gynecol **111**:778, 1971.
15. Judd HL, Lucas WE, Yen SSC: Amer J Obstet Gynecol **118**:793, 1974.
16. Calanog A, Sall S, Gordon GG, et al: Amer J Obstet Gynecol **124**:60, 1976.
17. Poortman J, Thijssen JHH, Schwartz F: J Clin Endocrinol Metab **37**:101, 1973.
18. Maroulis G, Abraham G: Obstet Gynecol **48**:150, 1976.
19. Abraham GE, Buster JE, Kyle FW, et al: J Clin Endocr Metab **37**:140, 1973.
20. Siiteri PK, MacDonald PC, in *Handbook of Physiology*, Greep RO, Astwood EB (eds.), Washington, DC, American Physiological Society, vol. II, part I, p. 615.
21. Baird DT, Uno A, Melby JC: J Endocrinol **45**:135, 1969.
22. Saez JJ, Morrera AM, Dazord A, et al: J Endocrinol **55**:41, 1972.
23. Brown JB, Falconer CWA, Strong JA: J Endocrinol **19**:52, 1959.
24. Barlow JJ, Emerson K, Saxena BN: N Engl J Med **280**:633, 1969.
25. Mattingly RF, Huang WY: Amer J Obstet Gynecol **103**:679, 1969.
26. Judd HL, Judd GE, Lucas WE, et al: J Clin Endocrinol Metab **39**:1020, 1974.
27. Greenblatt RB, Colle ML, Mahesh VB: Obstet Gynecol **47**:383, 1976.
28. Vermeulen A: J Clin Endocrinol Metab **42**:247, 1976.
29. Abraham GE, Maroulis GB: Obstet Gynecol **45**:271, 1975.
30. Steinach E, Kun H: Lancet **2**:845, 1937.
31. West CD, Dawast BL, Sarro SD, et al: J Biol Chem **218**:409, 1956.
32. MacDonald PC, Rombant RP, Siiteri PK: J Clin Endocrinol Metab **27**:1103, 1967.
33. Schindler AE, Ebert A, Fredrick E: J Clin Endocrinol Metab **35**:627, 1972.
34. Nimrod A, Ryan KJ: J Clin Endocrinol Metab **40**:367, 1975.
35. Judd HL, Lucas WE, Yen SSC: J Clin Endocrinol Metab **43**:272, 1976.
36. Rizkallah TH, Tovell HMM, Kelly WG: J Clin Endocrinol Metab **40**:1045, 1975.
37. Gurpide E, Angers M, Vande Wiele RL, et al: J Clin Endocrinol Metab **22**:935, 1962.
38. Marshall DH, Fearnley M, Holmes A, et al: in *Consensus on Menopause Research,* van Keep PA, Greenblatt RB, Albeaux-Fernet M (eds.), Baltimore, University Park Press, 1976, p. 100.
39. Edman CD, Hemsell DL, Siiteri PK, et al: Gynecol Invest **6**:23, 1975.
40. Siiteri PK, Schwarz BE, MacDonald PC: Gynecol Oncol **2**:228, 1974.
41. Urist MR: in *Bone as a Tissue*, Rohdahl K, Nicholson JR, Brown EM Jr (eds.), New York, McGraw-Hill, 1960, p. 126.
42. Albright F, Smith PH, Richardson AM: J Amer Med Ass **116**:2465, 1941.
43. Nordin BEC: Brit Med J **1**:571, 1971.
44. Aitken JM, Hoit DM, Lindsay R: Brit Med J **3**:515, 1973.
45. Heaney RP: NY State J Med **75**:1656, 1975.
46. Heaney RP: Clin Obstet Gynecol **19**:791, 1976.
47. Hernberg CA: Acta Endocrinol **34**:51, 1960.

48. Kannel WB, Barry P, Dawber TR: Proceedings, IV World Congress of Cardiology, Mexico City, p. 176.

49. Furman RH: in *Metabolic Effects of Gonadal Hormones and Contraceptive Steroids,* Salhanick HA, Kipnis DM, Vande Wiele RL (eds.), New York, Plenum Press, 1969, p. 246.

50. Pick R, Stamler J, Rodbard S, et al: Circulation **6:**276, 1952.

51. Stamler J, Pick R, Katz L, et al: in *Coronary Artery Disease*, Likoff W, Moyer JH (eds.), Hahneman Symposium on Coronary Heart Disease, 1963, p. 416.

52. Oliver MF, Boyd GS: Lancet **2:**499, 1961.

53. Mann JI, Inman WHW: Brit Med J **2:**245, 1975.

54. Kannel WB, Hjortland MC, McNamara PM: Ann Intern Med **85:**447, 1976.

55. Stern MP, Brown BW, Haskell WL, et al: J Amer Med Ass **235:**811, 1976.

Treatment of Menopause

John McLean Morris, M.D.

Considering the fact that approximately 27,000,000 women in the United States have undergone or are now undergoing menopause, it is surprising how little we really know about the process. With the loss of the ovarian follicular apparatus, there is a fall in estrogen, and of androgen and cyclic progesterone, and a rise in gonadotropin. But what is a hot flash? What is the physiologic mechanism that causes the presumed capillary dilatation and hyperhidrosis of the face, neck, and anterior chest wall? Why are women affected and not men? What is the basis for the concomitant insomnia or negative calcium balance?

Menopause may be a part of the aging process (median age at onset, about 51 years), but the symptoms should not be confused with those of aging. Declining libido, fatigue, wrinkles, decreased muscle tone, memory loss, and depression may also occur in the male. Menopause may also be induced by surgical removal of the ovaries or radiologic treatment ($\sim$ 1200 rads to the ovaries). Castration of the male or the XY female with testes (such as testicular feminization) does not usually result in significant hot flashes. The female to male transsexual, however, may develop menopausal symptoms postcastration that are uncontrolled with androgen administration.

The accompanying hormonal changes are obviously more abrupt, with more severe symptoms in surgically induced as compared to natural menopause, but a second significant difference is the fact that the postmenopausal ovary may continue to produce reduced amounts of androstenedione and testosterone. In some instances, the presence of the androgen unopposed by any estrogen may result in hirsutism, breast atrophy, or other signs of virilization. This is particularly true in the thin patient.

The obese patient is less likely to have significant menopausal symptoms, apparently related to the peripheral conversion by fat of androstenedione from adrenal or ovarian sources to estrone. However, the risk of many diseases in association with obesity, including not only endometrial cancer but also diabetes, hypertension, cerebrovascular accidents, and coronary disease, is such that while banning saccharin may reduce bladder cancer, it will doubtless increase death rates from other causes.

ROLE OF ESTROGENS

Estrogens alter mitotic activity at estrogen-binding sites. These sites include the pituitary, liver, bone, breast, uterus, and Müllerian and mesothelial epithelium. Estrogens are not carcinogens in the sense that coal tar derivatives and other mutants are, but with more mitoses, as with more automobiles, there may be more accidents. The kind of estrogen administered is not of importance: all appear to act in the same way. There is no evidence, for example, to support the hypothesis that estrone, Premarin, or diethylstilbestrol does anything harmful that any other estrogenic substance will not do. The dose and the duration of administration of estrogen are extremely important, as is the time in an individual's development at which the estrogen is given. When given after fertilization in the 5 days prior to implantation, estrogens can serve as contraceptives or, more correctly, interceptives. When given during uterine and vaginal organogenesis, they increase Müllerian mitotic activity and decrease the mitotic activity of the urogenital sinus area. This action results in adenosis of the exocervix and vagina. These glands may subsequently develop into cancer, but the term "transplacental carcinogenesis" is misleading. When given prior to puberty, estrogens and androgens may accelerate growth and secondary sexual development, to eventually cause premature epiphyseal closure and reduced stature. During reproductive life, they may inhibit ovulation. The effects at menopause will be the subject of this discussion.

RISKS OF HORMONAL REPLACEMENT

In 1974, the author discussed a paper presented by Smith at the District ACOG meeting in Los Angeles in which 48% of a series of patients with endometrial cancer were found to have taken estrogen, as compared with 17% in a control group (18). Because it has long been known that estrogens will increase the incidence of breast and uterine cancer in various animal species and that women with obesity or increased ovarian estrogen production tend to develop endometrial hyperplasia and carcinoma, these results did not appear particularly surprising. The author's impression was that our experience at Yale would tend to confirm these findings, depending to some extent on what group one uses for controls, but I correctly anticipated the media reaction.

The media create villains and heroes. At the moment estrogens are villains. The benefits of estrogen administration have attracted less attention than the risks, which are exaggerated by a national cancerphobia. The effect is unfortunate. Efforts to ban cancer have to date been unsuccessful, but nonexistent cancer risk in a nonexistent child has made abortion preferable to the morning-after pill in Washington.

Other statistical papers have described an increase in the incidence of endometrial cancer in the United States, using, among other sources, the Connecticut State Tumor Registry. The increase in Connecticut has all been in the earlier stages of the disease. The incidence of carcinoma in situ of the endometrium in Connecticut in 1970–4 (1.8/100,000 women) was double that of 1960–4 and of localized invasive disease (19.6/100,000 women) was nearly 20% greater, while the incidence of nonlocalized invasive disease (3.2/100,000 women) remained essentially unchanged in this period (13).

Perhaps the most significant figure in Connecticut is the reduction in uterine cancer death rates. The age-adjusted mortality rate from corpus carcinoma per 100,000 women has dropped from 8.2 in the 5-year period 1940–4 to 4.6 in 1960–4 and to 4.1 in the 1970–4 period.

It is important to recognize that the normal life-span of the disease may be 8–10 years or more. The median age at time of diagnosis of in situ carcinoma of the corpus in Connecticut (1960–74) was 52.5 years, of localized disease 60.3 years, and of patients with distant spread 65.1 years. At Yale, the mean age of patients with grade-1 tumors was 56 years, with grade-2 tumors was 60.5 years, and with grade-3 tumors was 64.3 years. Some of the increased incidence, therefore, may be the result of better medical practice, making earlier diagnosis with the use of such techniques as office suction biopsy. Picking up 8 years of the disease rather than 4 would double the incidence rate. The fact that the incidence of carcinoma in situ of the cervix in Connecticut increased from 4.0/100,000 women in 1950–4 to 28.8/100,000 women in 1970–4, with a decrease both in the incidence of invasive disease and in deaths from cervical cancer, is an illustration of such improved medical monitoring (11).

Nonetheless, there appears to be an increased risk of developing cancer of the uterus and breast in patients who have been taking exogenous estrogens. Approximately 40% of the endometrial cancers treated at Yale in recent years have been in patients taking exogenous estrogens. In a study from South Carolina, however, Underwood found that patients with endometrial cancer who had taken estrogen were younger (mean age of 57.2 years compared to 62.3 years in the nonestrogen cases), thinner, and had earlier lesions and better survival (97.6% at 5 years using corrected life tables) (19). This finding suggests that with exogenous estrogen, there may be more careful medical observation and earlier diagnosis and/or earlier induction of a tumor that is of lower-grade malignancy than its nonexogenously induced counterpart.

The question of thromboembolic and cardiovascular disorders is at present not settled, but to the risks that have been mentioned, another risk must be added. This is a risk that the legal profession has wished upon us. I am speaking of lawsuits. For example, a patient had an early carcinoma of the ovary removed at the age of 41. She was quite appropriately placed on estrogen by her physician. After taking hormones for 10 years, she sued him for a cancerphobia (plus weight gain and heavy breasts that caused pressure on her spine). The amount of damages she is seeking is half a million dollars.

BENEFITS OF HORMONAL REPLACEMENT

One benefit of hormonal replacement that does not exist is "feminine forever." There is no evidence that estrogens halt the development of the aging process in the ordinary sense of the word. No one can argue with the fact that hormones do relieve the symptoms of menopause. The most obvious and immediate benefit of exogenous estrogens is the relief of menopausal symptoms.

This benefit is illustrated in an excerpt of a letter from a patient:

"I stopped taking estrogen. . . . My hot flashes started again and got persistently more frequent. I began not to sleep and would wake every night around 5 a.m. Worse than those two things, was that I was becoming gradually more depressed and tired. In view of this, I filled the prescription that you gave me for estrogen, and will gladly take my chances with cancer—commonly known as living in the present."

Atrophy of the vaginal mucous membranes may be equally incapacitating because of severe vaginal dyspareunia. Quality of life is as important as quantity. But how does one do a statistical study on a sense of well-being?

What the patient does not notice until it is too late is calcium loss. Bone loss with age is well documented. The loss of bone mass in women is much more severe than in men and amounts to 1–3%/year at menopause. Significant osteoporosis is estimated to occur in about 25% of postmenopausal women (6).

It is usually discovered when x-rays are taken because of fractures or chronic back pain. The ratios of fractures in youth and middle age in women and men are essentially similar, but in the older age groups, reported female/male ratios for fractures of the hip are approximately 3:1, of the spine 4:1, and of the wrist 6–10:1 (Figure 1). The problem is a serious one, as reflected by the fact that in older women, the risk of hip fractures may reach 20% or more (3, 4, 9).

Various studies show that approximately 80% of hip fractures occur in patients over 60 and that 80–85% of this group are women. The mortality from hip fractures ranges between 4 and 32%. In 30 reported series, totaling 10,978 fractures, the combined mortality was 1450 (13.2%). Of 1114 cases reported by Alffram, 9% were dead in 1 month and 15% died within 3 months of the injury (3) (Figure 2).

There were 294 hip fractures treated in New Haven, Connecticut in a 1-year

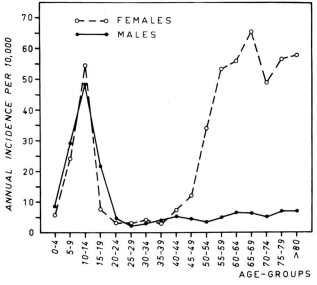

Figure 1. Incidence of fracture of the wrist shows the increase in older women. [Reprinted from Alffram et al. (4), J Bone Joint Surg **44A:**105, 1962.]

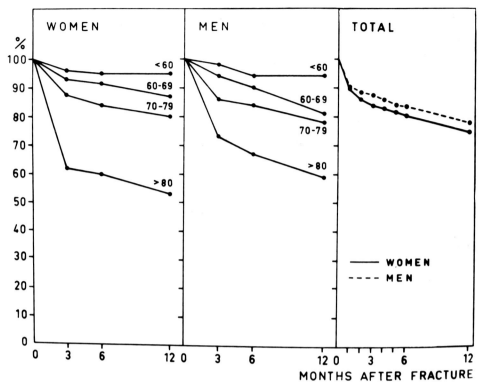

Figure 2. Survival rates 3, 6, and 12 months after hip fracture according to age and sex. [From Alffram (3).]

period beginning July 1, 1975. This figure compares with 68 cases of endometrial cancer during this period. The National Center for Health Statistics estimated that 184,000 hip fractures occurred in 1975 in the United States, of which more than 132,000 occurred in women. While the estimated annual death rate from hip fracture is considerably in excess of that from endometrial cancer, broken bones do not seem to strike the terror elicited by the word cancer, which to some is synonymous with death.

The problem of osteoporosis is a complicated one, and it involves many factors besides estrogens and androgens, including parathyroid hormone, vitamin D, exercise, calcium intake, fluoride, calcitonin, and, doubtless, many unknowns.

Albright's original work related osteoporosis to estrogen deficiency, because approximately 95% of the osteoporosis cases seen at Massachusetts General Hospital were postmenopausal women. He was further impressed by the finding of high calcium levels during the egg-laying cycle in birds and by Gardner and Pfeiffer's demonstration of the marked increase in bone density produced by estrin therapy in doves. Studies by Albright and coworkers showed that estrogen and androgen reverse the negative calcium balance of menopause. Osteoporosis could be halted but not reversed by estrogen administration. Vertebral deformity and loss of height could be arrested but not restored by estrogen administration (2, 10) (Figure 3).

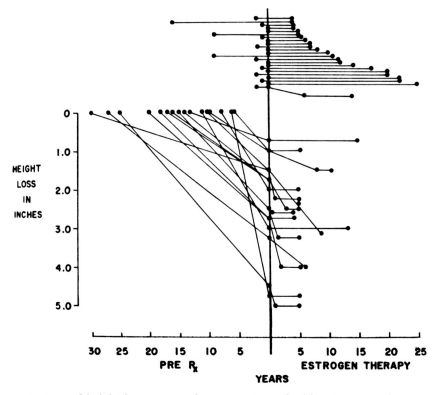

Figure 3. Loss of height in osteoporotic women treated with estrogen and untreated. [From Henneman and Wallach (10), Arch Intern Med **100:**715, copyright 1957 American Medical Association.]

These observations have been confirmed by so many others that charges of "unscientific studies" and "inadequate controls" seem ill-founded. The evidence is sufficiently conclusive that if a patient were put in the control group or given placebos in such a study and broke her hip or suffered a compression fracture of the spine, the researcher might have to do some soul-searching.

Whatever the roles of race, diet, exercise, and other factors may be, the increased bone resorption rates seen in menopause are reduced by estrogens and androgens.

In Canada, Meema et al. observed a significant difference in bone mineral mass between estrogen-treated and untreated menopausal women (15). Cortical bone thickness was considerably less in 33 untreated as compared with 20 hormone-treated castrates (14).

At the Mayo Clinic, Riggs et al. have demonstrated a uniformly beneficial effect of estrogen in reducing bone resorption in 11 osteoporotic women from elevated to normal levels (16) (Figure 4).

Davis and associates in Chicago, working with a photon absorption technique on bones of the hand, were able to show that bone loss was prevented or retarded in a group of patients with estrogen replacement since menopause and that bone density decreased much more rapidly in another group without estrogen replacement (6) (Figure 5).

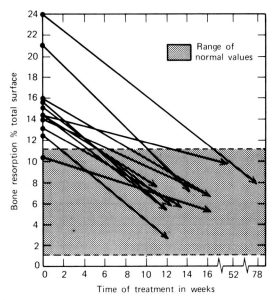

Figure 4. Effect of estrogen on bone resorption in 11 menopausal women. [From Riggs et al. (16). Used with copyright permission from The American Society of Clinical Investigation.]

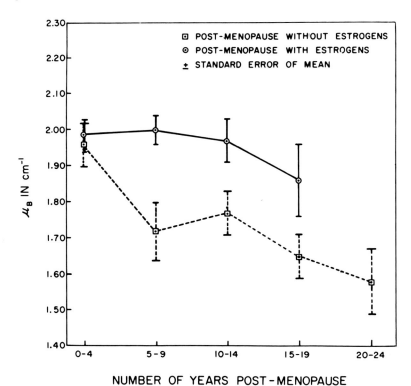

Figure 5. Bone density in the hand using photon absorption technique in estrogen-treated and untreated menopausal women. [From ME Davis, LH Lanzl, and AB Cox: The detection, prevention and retardation of menopausal osteoporosis, in *Osteoporosis,* US Barzel (ed), New York, Grune & Stratton, 1970, p. 140. Used by permission.]

A somewhat ruthless answer to the critics who demanded controls came from Scotland. Aitkin et al. demonstrated the mean yearly change in metacarpal mineral in oophorectomized women who received mestranol was significantly better than in controls given placebos when therapy was started within 3 years. In a smaller group of patients treated 6 years after oophorectomy, the differences noted were not statistically significant, suggesting that early hormone replacement is advisable (1). Lindsay and colleagues reported that placebo-"treated," oophorectomized patients followed for 5 years lost 2.7% of metacarpal mineral content per year compared to insignificant changes in bone mass in oophorectomized women treated daily with 24 μg of mestranol (12) (Figure 6).

TREATMENT OF MENOPAUSE

When is hormonal replacement therapy indicated?

1. It should not be given routinely to all menopausal patients or to prevent aging but should be prescribed in the presence of indications. The most common indication is menopausal symptoms. Hormonal replacement should be considered if hot flashes are frequent or severe enough to wake the patient at night or if vaginal discomfort interferes with marital relations.

2. The use of a wet smear obtained in the office at the time of the examination should be routine in such cases to establish the presence or absence of cornified cells, basal cells, or infection. Elaborate hormonal assays or cornification indices are not necessary and do not always correlate with the patient's symptomatology.

3. Replacement therapy should be started early. The most rapid bone loss occurs in the first years of estrogen withdrawal. Subsequent hormonal therapy, while preventing increase in osteoporosis, will not restore this loss.

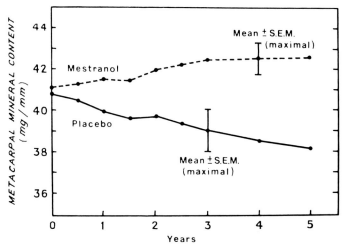

Figure 6. Mean metacarpal mineral content during 5-year follow-up after bilateral oophorectomy. [From Lindsay et al (12), Lancet 1:1038, 1976. Used by permission.]

4. Periodic checkups are necessary with breast and pelvic evaluation.

5. The patient should be instructed to report any bleeding. Should this phenomenon occur, hormonal therapy should be stopped for a period and office endometrial suction biopsy obtained. With persistent bleeding, a water-soluble hysterogram may be advisable or dilatation and curettage considered. Water-soluble hysterography is an insufficiently used technique in this country because of the erroneous fear that it will spread tumor. In our experience, this fear is not based on fact, and in more than 40% of cases, the procedure has revealed unexpected findings, particularly related to the size and location of the tumor (17).

6. Estrogen should be given in a cyclic fashion, at the lowest effective dose, and should be discontinued when no longer needed to control symptoms. This period varies widely from patient to patient and may amount to a few months or up to 10 years or more.

7. The major contraindications to exogenous estrogens are breast disease (mastalgia, cystic fibrosis), previous breast cancer, significant endometrial hyperplasia, or endometrial carcinoma. Patients with known phlebitis, migraine, or other such disorders may also be unable to take exogenous estrogen. Epidermoid carcinoma of the cervix is not a contraindication in the author's experience. In fact, in the younger patient with treated early endometrial cancer without evidence of recurrence at 6–12 months after hysterectomy, we may give estrogen to the severely symptomatic patient, the rationale being that the patient either is cured and therefore not at an increased risk or is not cured and therefore recurrence will ultimately manifest itself anyway.

What hormones should one give? Quantity and length of administration of estrogen are important. The particular estrogen employed is of little significance. All bind to the same estrogen receptors, the competition for the binding site being almost identical to the uterotrophic, and thus estrogenic, activity. Stilbenes are the least expensive estrogens to make, but many patients are frightened when they see the word diethylstilbestrol on a prescription. There is only one clinical difference between stilbenes and steroidal estrogens, namely, that the former darken the nipple areola and labial epithelium. Ethynyl estradiol, chlorotrianisene, and various esterified or conjugated estrogens are available alone or in combination with androgens, tranquilizers, minerals, or vitamins. Some preparations will occasionally produce nausea, but conjugated estrogens seem to be well tolerated by most patients. Federal Drug Administration restrictions would make it essentially impossible to change the 0.625 mg dose to 0.5 or 0.7 mg, but one only has to look through *Physicians Desk Reference* and see the number of 0.625 and 1.25 mg estrogen preparations to recognize the sheeplike quality of man, even in supposedly scientific areas. "The dawn of a new age" and new "natural" hormone products are similar to older preparations in their effects.

Basically, estrogen should be given in a cyclic fashion and in as low a dose and for as short a period as possible. It is easier to stop medication the first 5–7 days each month only because the 3 week-on and 1 week-off regimen is harder for the patient to follow. It requires 4–5 days for the pills to take effect and a similar period for the effect to wear off. If no symptoms appear on the fifth to seventh days of abstinence, it may be possible to reduce or discontinue the hormone. Often, dose reduction is accomplished best by taking a pill every other day or two or three times a week.

Should one add progesterone? Progestational agents can cause marked regression of endometrial cancer and of metastatic lesions. Progesterone has been shown to lower endometrial estradiol receptor levels and increase estradiol 17β-dehydrogenase activity, converting estradiol to the less active estrone. On the other hand, studies by Griffiths et al. showed that addition of gestagens to estrogen administration in castrated rabbits did not reduce the incidence of endometrial cancer (8). Some also apparently believe that sequential estrogen and progesterone administration is associated with an increased incidence of endometrial cancer in young women.

The major reasons not to add progesterone are that it will produce withdrawal bleeding in patients on estrogen, causing emotional stress and unnecessary endometrial biopsy or curettage, and that progesterone raises basal body temperature for reasons unknown, possibly due to changes in the carbohydrate metabolic pathways, and may cause a feeling of fatigue, decrease in libido, and loss of the sense of well-being that the menopausal treatment is directed toward. The disadvantages would appear to outweigh the possible reduced cancer risk advantage, but no scientific study has yet been performed to show that the endometrial cancer risk is actually reduced.

What about the addition of androgen, since testosterone levels also decline at menopause? Estrogens and androgens may have similar or synergistic effects in some areas, such as in reversing the negative calcium balance in osteoporosis. In other areas, such as the breast, they may have opposite effects. A man without the suppressive effect of his testosterone will develop gynecomastia (e.g., in Klinefelter's syndrome or testicular feminization). Testosterone will reverse the carcinogenic effects of estrogen on breast tumor development in experimental animals (7). The effect of androgens on the endometrium has been studied very little, but androgens may be of value in the treatment of endometriosis. While it is doubtful that androgens would reduce endometrial cancer incidence, this question is still unresolved. Androgens will, however:

· supplement the beneficial effect of estrogens in preventing osteoporosis
· reverse some of the harmful effects of estrogen on the breast, including painful engorgement, or, in animal experiments, cancer risk
· increase libido
· increase a sense of well-being and "get up and go."

The addition of androgen may be advisable in patients who have undergone surgical or radiologic castration because of the loss of ovarian production of testosterone. It may also be beneficial in the treatment of other menopausal patients, particularly if breast problems exist or with loss of libido or decreased sense of well-being. It is contraindicated in the patient who complains of the hirsutism or breast atrophy that may accompany the menopause.

The dosage (usually oral methyltestosterone given in combined tablets with estrogen) should be in the 2.5 or 5.0 mg/day range. Virilization will be almost invariably noted if the patient continues for any period of time on a 10.0 mg/day dose. Even the 5.0 mg dose will sometimes cause acne, increased facial hair, or breast atrophy, and 2.5 mg may be preferable.

The younger oophorectomized patient may require relatively high doses of estrogen (1.25–2.5 mg of conjugated estrogens) for a protracted period and will usually achieve better results with the addition of some androgen. To quote from a medical endocrinologist serving as her own control postoophorectomy comparing estrogens with testosterone (red) and without:

> I would say I feel "normal," that is full of pep and able to do my usual 16 hour day without batting an eye on your red pill. Libido fine, a bit euphoric. On the yellow and orange varieties I don't have any symptoms, but I feel draggy and can't work at night. I just don't have my usual pep and bounce. On no pills I have both sweats and hot flashes and feel what I would describe as "a bit shaky." This sounds pretty crocky, but I wouldn't want to make a major decision and seem to get mad and irritable without provocation . . . . So if you have no objections, is it okay to take a red pill a day forever?

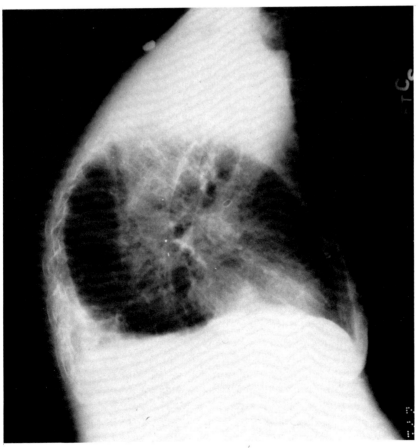

Figure 7. Sixty-one-year-old patient with partial paralysis related to compression fractures of the spine. Note osteoporosis of vertebral bodies. Patient is a permanent invalid.

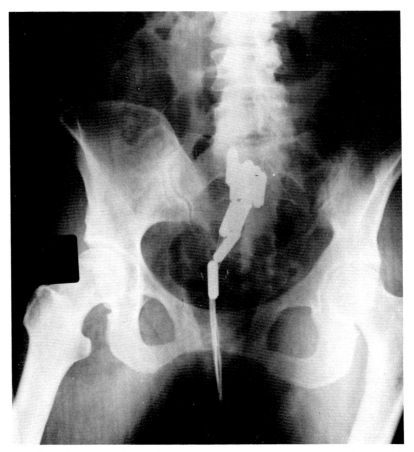

Figure 8. Sixty-eight-year-old patient on exogenous estrogens for 23 years. Radium packing is in place for endometrial carcinoma. Note bone density of vertebral bodies and femoral necks. Patient is free of disease.

Byrd et al., in a series of 1016 hysterectomized patients treated with estrogen and followed for 14,318 patient-years, found a decrease in expected deaths from all causes (54 vs. 149 expected), including heart disease and cerebrovascular accidents. Fractures of the forearm numbered 23 rather than the expected 40. Breast cancer incidence was slightly increased (33 vs. 24 expected), but deaths from breast cancer were less, probably because of the earlier diagnosis in the individuals under observation. Deaths from all cancers numbered 23 as compared with 29 expected (5).

Thus, both quantity and quality of life may be improved by exogenous hormone replacement. Early endometrial cancer has the best cure rate of any intraabdominal or gynecologic cancer. One can usually treat early cases successfully. However, medicine has little to offer for the patient partially paralyzed by compression fractures of an osteoporotic spine (Figures 7 & 8). Estrogens have an important place in therapy.

REFERENCES

1. Aitken JM, Hart DM, Lindsay R: Oestrogen replacement therapy for prevention of osteoporosis after oophorectomy. Brit Med J **3:**515, 1973.

2. Albright F, Bloomberg E, Smith PH: Postmenopausal osteoporosis. Trans Ass Amer Physicians **55:**298, 1940.

3. Alffram PA: An epidemiologic study of cervical and intertrochanteric fractures of the femur in an urban population. Acta Orthopaed Scand Suppl **65:**1, 1964.

4. Alffram PA, Bauer GCH: Epidemiology of fractures of the forearm. J Bone Joint Surg **44A:**105, 1962.

5. Byrd BF Jr, Burch JC, Vaughn WK: The impact of long term estrogen support of the hysterectomy—a report of 1016 cases. Ann Surg **185:**574, 1977.

6. Davis ME, Lanzl LH, Cox AB: The detection, prevention and retardation of menopausal osteoporosis, in *Osteoporosis*, Barzel US (ed.), New York, Grune & Stratton, 1970, p. 140.

7. Gardner WU: Tumors in experimental animals receiving steroid hormones. Surgery **16:**8, 1944.

8. Griffiths CT, Craig JM, Kistner RW, et al: Effect of castration, estrogen and timed progestins on induced endometrial carcinoma in the rabbit. Gynecol Oncol **3:**259, 1973.

9. Heaney RP: Estrogens and postmenopausal osteoporosis. Clin Obstet Gynecol **19:**791, 1976.

10. Henneman PH, Wallach S: A review of the prolonged use of estrogens and androgens in postmenopausal and senile osteoporosis. Arch Intern Med **100:**715, 1957.

11. Laskey PW, Meigs JW, Flannery JT: Uterine cervical carcinoma in Connecticut, 1935–1973: evidence for two classes of invasive disease. J Nat Cancer Inst **57:**1037, 1976.

12. Lindsay R, Aitken JM, Anderson JB, et al: Long-term prevention of postmenopausal osteoporosis by oestrogen. Lancet **1:**1038, 1976.

13. Marrett LD, Elwood JM, Meigs JW, et al: Recent trends in the incidence and mortality of cancer of the uterine corpus in Connecticut. Gynecol Oncol **6:**183, 1978.

14. Meema HE, Meema S: Prevention of postmenopausal osteoporosis by hormone treatment of the menopause. Can Med Ass J **99:**248, 1968.

15. Meema S, Bunker ML, Meema HE: Preventive effect of estrogen on postmenopausal bone loss. Arch Intern Med **135:**1436, 1975.

16. Riggs BL, Jowsey J, Kelly PH, et al: Effect of sex hormones on bone in primary osteoporosis. J Clin Invest **48:**1065, 1969.

17. Schwartz PE, Kohorn EI, Knowlton AH, et al: Routine use of hysterography in endometrial carcinoma and postmenopausal bleeding. Obstet Gynecol **45:**378, 1975.

18. Smith DC, Prentice R, Thompson DJ, et al: Association of exogenous estrogen and endometrial carcinoma. N Engl J Med **11:**64, 1975.

19. Underwood PB Jr: Unpublished data.

DISCUSSION

Question: Has any work been performed on osteoporosis in castrated males?

Dr. Morris: I don't know of any reports relating to your question. It has been established that males also lose bone mass as they age. In women, however, this loss is so much more rapid that I think it is a different phenomenon. Birds will be pleased to note that females have much stronger bone structure than do male birds, and this difference is thought to be related to the egg-laying cycle and estrogens. I feel that while there are many factors involved, the loss of steroidal hormones plays a definite role, and I suspect that this would be the case in castrated men. Males who are castrated are very apt to receive estrogens for prostatic cancer or as replacement hormonal therapy.

Question: You listed the risk of cancer of the breast as a contraindication to estrogen therapy. Do you have any evidence that estrogen contributes to cancer of the breast?

Dr. Morris: The first evidence is that 40 years of animal experiments show an increase of breast cancer incidence in animals receiving estrogen. In a recent study (Hoover R, Gray LA Sr, Cole P, et al: N Engl J Med **295**:401, 1976), a slightly increased incidence was demonstrated. One might ask the important question: "Is it the same cancer or is it a more benign cancer?" I think that the cancer might be caused by estrogen or we may be detecting it earlier. I would seriously argue with the statistician who says that there won't be an increase or there hasn't been an increase.

Menopausal Estrogens and Endometrial Cancer

Noel S. Weiss, M.D.

Although estrogen preparations have been available since the early 1930s, it has only been during the past one to two decades that their use has gained widespread acceptance among American physicians and their menopausal patients. From the mid-1960s to mid-1970s alone, the rate of menopausal estrogen use increased several-fold in this country (1). The increase has varied from place to place; the data available suggest that estrogens are now generally more popular in the western United States than in the eastern part of the country (2–5).

Preliminary data from a recent sample survey of 35–74-year-old female residents of King and Pierce County (Washington), in which respondents were asked detailed questions regarding hormone intake, can be used to illustrate the magnitude and determinants of estrogen exposure (Table 1). Among the 541 women interviewed, 380 stated that their menstrual periods had stopped one or more years previously. In this group, 50.8% had used noncontraceptive estrogens for at least one year. Women who had undergone a surgical menopause reported estrogen use more commonly than did women with spontaneous menopause (67.2 vs. 36.5%). Postmenopausal women under the age of 60 had more often taken estrogens than had those over 60, a reflection of the increasing popularity of these agents in recent years.

The high percentage of users is a tribute to the perceived benefits of estrogens to menopausal women. Several of the benefits seem to be real ones, for example, relief of acute menopausal symptoms (6) and retardation of osteoporosis (7), so that a decision to not initiate or to discontinue estrogen treatment due to possible adverse effects should have a solid basis. Another implication of the present high prevalence of estrogen use by menopausal women is that even small relative benefits and risks relating to their use will be magnified in terms of the effect on the health of this segment of the population.

EXOGENOUS ESTROGENS AND ENDOMETRIAL CANCER: IS THE RELATIONSHIP A CAUSAL ONE?

A cause of a disease can be considered as anything of which it can be said that had it not been present, some cases of the disease would not have occurred. This

Table 1. Estrogen Use in a Random Sample of 380 King and Pierce County Postmenopausal Women

	Percentage of Users for ≥ 1 Year
All	50.8
Spontaneous menopause	36.5
Surgical menopause	67.2
< 60 years old	61.6
≥ 60 years old	39.5

kind of pragmatic definition is probably the most appropriate for purposes of deciding on preventive action; it allows for both multiple causes of a disease and for failure of the disease to follow inevitably the putative cause. Alcoholic intoxication is generally accepted as a cause of automobile accidents, yet it is possible to be intoxicated and not have an accident or to have an accident and not be intoxicated. As long as some accidents can be prevented by sobriety, though, the above definition of cause is met.

By this definition, estrogens are almost certainly a cause of endometrial cancer. Although the definitive studies that could shed light on this question (large, randomized trials with long-term followup) have never been performed, the nonexperimental evidence that has been assembled is convincing.

1. Pattern of occurrence
   Incidence rates of endometrial cancer in the United States, after many years of stability, rose sharply soon after the rapid rise in estrogen use among American menopausal women (8) (Table 2). In contrast, endometrial cancer rates in England, where noncontraceptive estrogen use has been much less common, are lower than in the United States and have not increased during the same period (9).

2. Studies of individual subjects
   Five recent studies showed that menopausal women with endometrial cancer had a greater exposure to exogenous estrogens than did controls (2, 10–13). The incidence in users was estimated to be three to 10 times that in nonusers. Two other case control studies failed to find such a relationship (14, 15), but because the controls in these studies were drawn from women with conditions related to estrogen use (e.g., uterine bleeding), their results should be given far less weight. Additional evidence comes from studies of endometrial hyperplasia. Estrogen use has been found to predispose to this condition (16), and women with hyperplasia have an increased risk of carcinoma (17, 18).

3. Other evidence
   a. Conditions in which endogenous estrogen levels are elevated (e.g., obesity)

Table 2. Annual Uterine Corpus Cancer Incidence Rates[a] in Selected Areas of the United States by Year, 1969–73 [From Weiss et al. (8). By permission of *The New England Journal of Medicine.*]

Area	Year				
	1969	1970	1971	1972	1973
Connecticut[b]	18.0	19.2	21.8	23.0	25.9
Hawaii	26.6	21.1	23.8	23.2	35.6
Los Angeles County[c]	[d]	[d]	[d]	34.6	33.5
New Mexico	10.2	13.0	16.8	20.7	17.9
Oregon[bef]	27.9	24.2	30.4	36.2	[d]
San Francisco Bay area	24.9	27.9	30.9	35.2	40.3
Seattle-Tacoma	[d]	[d]	[d]	[d]	45.6[g]
Utah[e]	[d]	19.3	21.6	29.9	23.9

[a] Per 100,000 women, standardized to the age distribution of the 1970 United States population; excludes adenocarcinoma in situ, unless otherwise indicated.

[b] Rates include those for in situ cancers.

[c] Whites only (excluding Mexican-Americans).

[d] Data unavailable for that year.

[e] Intercensal estimates of population size not available for this area; 1970 population used as basis for rates in all years.

[f] Incidence of uterine adenocarcinoma (both corpus and cervix).

[g] Annual rate estimated from data from first 6 months of 1974.

or are not countered by progesterone secretion (e.g., polycystic ovarian disease) predispose to endometrial cancer (19).

b. Use of noncontraceptive estrogens in two circumstances other than the menopause, gonadal agenesis and breast cancer, leads to an increased incidence of endometrial cancer (20–22).

c. Proliferation of cells is a necessary condition for carcinogenesis (23), and endometrial proliferation is a prominent effect of estrogenic hormones.

Do we have enough evidence to infer that menopausal estrogens are a cause of endometrial cancer? The parallel between this association and that of prenatal diethylstilbestrol (DES) exposure with vaginal adenocarcinoma, in which a causal relationship is generally conceded, may be of help in answering this question. Almost all of the human evidence that relates DES to vaginal adenocarcinoma comes from retrospective data on the high frequency of exposure among cases relative to controls (24, 25) and from the rising (though still low) incidence of the disease after the introduction of DES therapy in pregnancy (26). Follow-up studies of DES-exposed girls have, in fact, generally been negative (27–29), again due to the rarity of the disease. The latter studies do seem to indicate that prenatal DES exposure is not a direct cause of adenocarcinoma but, rather, often leads to a benign condition, vaginal adenosis, which, in the presence of other, unknown factors, can occasionally be associated with cancer.

All of the above is the same kind of evidence that links menopausal estrogens to endometrial cancer (rising incidence rates, strongly positive case control studies, induction of a nonmalignant lesion that precedes the development of cancer) and argues strongly that this link is also a causal one.

CAN ESTROGENS BE USED BY MENOPAUSAL WOMEN IN SUCH A WAY AS TO MINIMIZE THE INCREASED RISK OF ENDOMETRIAL CANCER?

As cited earlier, menopausal women who use noncontraceptive estrogen preparations have, on the average, a three- to 10-fold increased incidence of endometrial cancer relative to estrogen nonusers. Judging from the evidence gathered to date, the magnitude of this increased incidence can be modified to some extent by the way in which estrogens are taken:

a. Dose
    In each of the three studies that examined the question, the estrogen-endometrial cancer association is strongest for the highest strength preparations (2, 12, 13). The incidence of endometrial cancer in the woman who has used the lower doses, such as .625 mg. of conjugated estrogens or less, is still greater than that in the nonuser, but now by a factor of approximately 1.5 to 5.0.

b. Duration of use
    All of the studies agree that the longer a woman uses noncontraceptive estrogens, the greater her risk of endometrial cancer (2, 11–13). The woman who has taken estrogens for only a few years has an approximately 1.2- to 4.5-fold increased risk of the disease. Whether one year's use or less increases endometrial cancer incidence is unknown: few women in the studies to date have had such brief exposure.

c. Estrogen-free intervals each month
    Only two of the studies have examined the relation of cycling of estrogen use to increased risk (2, 12), and the results are inconclusive.

d. Addition of progestagen to the regimen
    Because periodic progestagen administration produces endometrial regression and sloughing, it might be expected that this mode of therapy would not increase cancer risk. Progestagen use was rare in the subjects of the five case control studies and could not be evaluated. Preliminary results from a newer study in which a progestagen was added to the estrogen regimen of menopausal women indicate that these patients experienced a normal incidence of endometrial cancer (30), but much more information is needed.

From the foregoing, it is probable that if the current recommendation (31) for menopausal estrogen use (low dose, short duration) is followed, the increased risk of endometrial cancer will be less than the average increase found in most of the recent studies. How closely this risk will approach that of nonusers is unknown, as is the benefit this regimen provides for osteoporosis prevention, and so on. The periodic addition of progestagen is a therapeutic modality supported on theoretical grounds, but its actual effect on endometrial cancer risk and acceptability to menopausal women is unknown. The direction of further research in this field, then, is clear, but for the present time, a good deal of uncertainty remains regarding the long-term consequences of these drugs.

ROLE OF CASE CONTROL STUDIES IN ETIOLOGIC RESEARCH

Case control studies are defined as those in which persons with a given attribute, commonly a disease, are compared to persons without that attribute regarding various antecedent exposures or characteristics. The hope, as in all epidemiologic research, is that substantial differences between ill and well persons will emerge that might suggest the causes of that illness.

If a case control study were the only source of data bearing on a particular question, it would be of little value. Patients with cancer report weight loss more commonly than do healthy men and women, yet it would be ludicrous to think that this type of "finding" suggests cause and effect. On the other hand, when incorporated with basic biologic and clinical knowledge and other epidemiologic observations, the results from case control studies can be very helpful in trying to infer a causal connection. One reason for the relatively great impact of the recent case control studies of endometrial cancer (2, 10–13), apart from the striking relationship they found, was that in conjunction with everything else known about estrogens and the endometrium, an association between estrogens and endometrial cancer made sense.

To the nonepidemiologist, there is something unaesthetic about case control studies: after all, why look for an association in this backward sort of way? Unfortunately, a choice of research strategies is usually not present. As indicated earlier, without case control studies, we would still be waiting for someone to follow-up enough DES-exposed daughters to find the link with vaginal adenocarcinoma. Apart from this, both retrospective (case control) and prospective (cohort) studies are really able to arrive at the same measure of association (32). Needless to say, both types of study can provide erroneous results through improper design and/or analysis. Subjects must be comparable, either through their selection or by adjustment in the analysis, and the method of measurement of exposure (case control study) or disease (cohort study) should be as unbiased and as accurate as possible. Nonetheless, when performed accurately, the two types of studies should be expected to yield similar results, as indeed they have in areas where both have been employed (33, 34).

REFERENCES

1. Pharmaceutical Preparations, Except Biologicals, 1973 [U.S. Bureau of the Census Current Industrial Reports, Series 17a-28G(73)-1]. Washington, DC, U.S. Government Printing Office, 1975.
2. Mack TM, Pike MC, Henderson BE, et al: Estrogens and endometrial cancer in a retirement community. N Engl J Med **294**:1262, 1976.
3. Pfeffer RI, Van DenNoort S: Estrogen use and stroke risk in postmenopausal women. Amer J Epidemiol **103**:445, 1976.

4. Nomura A, Comstock GC: Benign breast tumor and estrogenic hormones: a population-based retrospective study. Amer J Epidemiol **103**:439, 1976.

5. Rosenberg L, Armstrong B, Jick H: Myocardial infarction and estrogen therapy in postmenopausal women. N Engl J Med **294**:1256, 1976.

6. Coope J, Thompson JM, Poller L: Effects of "natural estrogen" replacement therapy on menopausal symptoms and blood clotting. Brit Med J **4**:139, 1975.

7. Lindsay R, Hart DM, Aitken JM: Long-term prevention of postmenopausal osteoporosis by estrogen. Lancet **1**:1038, 1976.

8. Weiss NS, Szekely DR, Austin DF: Increasing incidence of endometrial cancer in the United States. N Engl J Med **294**:1259, 1976.

9. Doll R, Kinlen LJ, Skegg DCG: Incidence of endometrial carcinoma. Lancet **1**:1071, 1976.

10. Smith DC, Prentice R, Thompson DJ, et al: Association of exogenous estrogen and endometrial carcinoma. N Engl J Med **293**:1164, 1975.

11. Ziel HK, Finkle WD: Increased risk of endometrial carcinoma among users of conjugated estrogens. N Engl J Med **293**:1167, 1975.

12. McDonald TW, Annegers JF, O'Fallon WM, et al: Exogenous estrogen and endometrial carcinoma: case-control and incidence study. Amer J Obstet Gynecol **127**:572, 1977.

13. Gray LA, Christopherson WM, Hoover RN: Estrogens and endometrial carcinoma. Obstet Gynecol **49**:385, 1977.

14. Horwitz RI, Feinstein AR: New methods of sampling and analysis to remove bias in case-control research: no association found for estrogens and endometrial cancer. Paper presented at Society for Epidemiologic Research 10th Anniversary Meeting, June 1977.

15. Dunn LJ, Bradbury JT: Endocrine factors in endometrial carcinoma: a preliminary report. Amer J Obstet Gynecol **97**:465, 1967.

16. Pacheco JC, Kempers RD: Etiology of postmenopausal bleeding. Obstet Gynecol **32**:40, 1968.

17. Campbell PE, Barter RA: The significance of atypical endometrial hyperplasia. J Obstet Gynecol Brit Common **68**:668, 1961.

18. Vellios F: Endometrial hyperplasias, precursors of endometrial carcinoma. Pathol Annu **7**:201, 1972.

19. MacDonald PC, Siiteri PK: The relationship between the extraglandular production of estrone and the occurrence of endometrial neoplasia. Gynecol Oncol **2**:259, 1974.

20. Cutler BS, Forbes AP, Ingersoll FM, et al: Endometrial carcinoma after stilbestrol therapy in gonadal dysgenesis. N Engl J Med **287**:628, 1972.

21. McCarroll AM, Montgomery DAD, Harley JMG, et al: Endometrial cancer after cyclical estrogen-progestogen therapy for Turner's syndrome. Brit J Obstet Gynecol **82**:421, 1975.

22. Hoover R, Fraumeni JF, Everson R, et al: Cancer of the uterine corpus after hormonal treatment for breast cancer. Lancet **1**:885, 1976.

23. Ryser HJP: Chemical carcinogenesis. N Engl J Med **285**:721, 1971.

24. Herbst AL, Ulfelder H, Poskanzer DC: Adenocarcinoma of the vagina. N Engl J Med **284**:878, 1971.

25. Greenwald P, Barlow JJ, Nasca PC, et al: Vaginal cancer after maternal treatment with synthetic estrogens. N Engl J Med **285**:390, 1971.

26. Herbst AL, Cole P, Colton T, et al: Age-incidence and risk of diethylstilbestrol-related clear cell adenocarcinoma of the vagina and cervix. Amer J Obstet Gynecol **128**:43, 1977.

27. Lanier HP, Noller KL, Decker DG, et al: Cancer and stilbestrol: a followup of 1719 persons exposed to estrogens in utero and born 1943–59. Mayo Clin Proc **48**:793, 1973.

28. Herbst AL, Poskanzer DC, Robboy SJ, et al: Prenatal exposure to stilbestrol: a prospective comparison of exposed female offspring with unexposed controls. N Engl J Med **292**:334, 1975.

29. Bibbo M, Gill WB, Azizi F, et al: Followup study of male and female offspring of DES-exposed mothers. Obstet Gynecol **49**:1, 1977.

30. Gambrell RD: Estrogens, progestogens and endometrial cancer. J Repro Med **18**:301, 1977.

31. Estrogen replacement therapy, ACOG Tech Bull **43,** 1976.

32. MacMahon B, Pugh TF: *Epidemiology: Principles and Methods.* Boston, Little, Brown and Company, 1970.
33. Doll R, Hill AB: Smoking and carcinoma of the lung. Brit Med J **2:**739, 1950.
34. Doll R, Peto R: Mortality in relation to smoking: 20 years' observations on male British doctors. Brit Med J **2:**1525, 1976.

DISCUSSION

Question: Are mortality figures for endometrial cancer increasing in relation to incidence figures?

Dr. Weiss: It's almost impossible to make any reliable assessment, either now or in the past. When we work with mortality data, we are dealing with death certificate assessments of disease. For many years in this country, and even up to now, the cause of death is listed only as uterine cancer, and whether it is a cervical cancer or endometrial cancer is uncertain. Since we also know that the incidence and mortality of cervical cancer are declining in the United States, if some of these tumors are falsely listed as uterine cancer, it makes the whole thing really messy. I believe, however, that we will not really see much of any mortality increase to correspond to the current increase in incidence, because endometrial cancers are local and low grade in the majority of cases, and those that seem to be related to estrogen use are on the even lower side of the spectrum.

Question: Do you have more specific data on the epidemiology of estrogen usage in terms of who receives estrogen? Of your 50% of women is there any difference constitutionally or socioeconomically between the 50% who had estrogen and the 50% who did not receive it?

Dr. Weiss: Correct, there are differences. In our studies, which we will be analyzing in more detail soon, there are indications that if you have hot flashes, you are a lot more likely to be receiving estrogens. If you're more highly educated, you are more likely to use estrogens, but not if you're over 60 years of age. In older women, it doesn't seem to make a difference, but if you are in your 50s or late 40s and highly educated, you are very likely to enter this drug regimen.

Question: In all of the papers that have described the association of the estrogens and endometrial cancer, one of the major discrepancies has been that there has really not been much pathologic analysis or review of the pathologic findings in the original slides. Several review papers have demonstrated that many of the patients have hyperplasia and not cancer. Can you give us an update on the various studies?

Dr. Weiss: This is the area in which many people have questions. I think that this problem can be approached in two ways. One is what we have been doing in the Seattle area, where you know there is evidence of increased incidence. We have had a single pathologist review every slide in the whole county of endometrial cancer during the first 6 months of 1975. We found, indeed, that there is much variation from standard criteria. We found about 20% of cases that were not really cancers by strict criteria. If you take those 20% away, there is still an enormously increased incidence in our area compared to what it was five years ago. Even better are the data soon to be published from a study in southern California, in which three very well-known pathologists read all of the slides on their studies and threw out those for which the consensus was not cancer. These workers have now recomputed the relative risk for the association between estrogen and cancer, using only the certified cancer patients, and that estimate was identical to their first figure (Gordon J, Reagan JW, Finkle WD, et al: N Engl J Med **297**:570, 1977).

Dr. Silverberg: As a pathologist, I might just point out that many people have criticized the endometrial carcinoma studies for this reason. Overdiagnosis of hyperplasias as carcinomas is certainly not limited to the endometrium. Similar data have been published for lymphomas, melanomas, mammary and many other types of cancer, so it's certainly not limited to the endometrium, although we probably would agree that the endometrium is one of the most difficult areas in which to make a definitive diagnosis.

Postmenopausal Estrogens and Endometrial Cancer: Clinicopathologic Correlations

Alexander Miller, M.D.

Dennis Mullen, M.D.

Jack A. Faraci, M.D.

Edgar L. Makowski, M.D.

Steven G. Silverberg, M.D.

The controversy surrounding the development of endometrial cancer in women receiving exogenous estrogen hormone has waxed and waned since these drugs were first developed in the late 1930s. As early as 1940, Allen (1) and Geist and Solmon (2) cautioned about the possible carcinogenic action on the breast and uterus of these compounds. The excellent review of Knab (3) details the historical background, biochemistry, and the recent clinical trials that have rekindled the interest in this problem.

Smith et al. (4) and Ziel and Finkle (5) in December 1975 published two studies with far-reaching effects. Subsequently, other case control studies have been published with data supporting the theory that there is an increased risk of developing endometrial cancer in women receiving exogenous estrogens (6–9). Ziel and Finkle studied 94 patients and showed a risk ratio increasing from 5.6 to 12.9 with duration of exposure. Smith et al. retrospectively studied 317 patients and reported a 4.5 times greater risk in the group receiving hormone therapy. These studies have been severely criticized for several reasons, the most important being poor choice of controls (10, 11). In the series of Smith et al., the controls were women with other gynecologic malignancies, usually cervical, a population known to have exactly opposite risk factors to those of endometrial carcinoma. Second, the lack of critical pathologic review has been considered a source of bias.

Supported in part by Grants CA-17060, CA-21878, and CA-15823
from the National Cancer Institute.

35

Since recent data (12) have shown that there is, in fact, a real increase in the incidence of this lesion in this country, and considering the longstanding known relationship between endogenous estrogen and endometrial cancer (13–15), we decided to approach the problem from a slightly different viewpoint. The material presented is a preliminary report on the first 114 patients in a cooperative study between the University of Colorado School of Medicine and Colorado Regional Cancer Center in Denver and Rush Medical School in Chicago.

Postmenopausal women diagnosed as having endometrial carcinoma between 1965 and 1975 were evaluated for several clinical and pathologic variables (Tables 1 & 2). The clinical and pathologic materials were collected and evalu-

Table 1.   Clinical Factors Evaluated

Prior estrogen use
Diabetes
Hypertension
Obesity
Parity
Years postmenopausal
Duration of symptoms
Clinical stage

Table 2.   Pathologic Factors Evaluated

Histologic grade
Histologic type
Concomitant hyperplasia
Presence of ciliated cells in tumor
Presence of clear cells in tumor
Presence of lymphoid infiltrate
Myometrial invasion
Vascular invasion

ated independently to eliminate bias. The tumors were critically reviewed histopathologically to eliminate all borderline lesions, such as adenomatous and atypical hyperplasias. All questionable lesions were discarded, as were cases in which a reliable history relating to hormone usage was not available. The tumors were graded as described by Gompel and Silverberg (16), and the FIGO staging system was used. No attempt was made to determine risk ratio or incidence in the populations represented. The purpose of this initial evaluation was to determine if a subpopulation could be identified, either by clinical or pathologic characteristics, that was related to exogenous hormone therapy.

Table 3 indicates the prevalence of clinical or chemical diabetes mellitus, hypertension, and obesity among the patients who had and had not received exogenous estrogen. In each category, the prevalence was significantly lower among the patients who had received estrogen. These findings confirm those of

Table 3. Prevalence of Diabetes, Hypertension, and
Obesity in Postmenopausal Endometrial Carcinoma
Patients With and Without Prior Estrogen Exposure

	No Estrogen	Estrogen
Diabetic	23/75	4/39
Hypertensive	32/75	9/39
Obese	44/66[a]	12/30[a]
	(p < 0.001 for each variable)	

[a] Stature unknown for nine of each set.

Smith et al. (4) with respect to obesity and hypertension and are also similar to
our data concerning obesity in endometrial cancer patients under 40 years of age
who had received Oracon, a sequential oral contraceptive (reported later in this
volume).

The differences between the estrogen users and nonusers were also significant
with respect to parity (Table 4), showing less of a tendency to nulliparity or low
parity among estrogen users. Again, these data are similar to those obtained in
our oral contraceptive study. Although the differences are less striking here, this
is probably a function of the fact that oral contraceptive users would be expected
to be multiparous as an indication for taking the medication, whereas no such
bias should exist for postmenopausal patients receiving estrogenic compounds.

The explanation for the lower prevalence of constitutional risk factors in
endometrial cancer patients who had received exogenous hormones is unknown.
Smith and colleagues (4) concluded that "this observation invites speculation
about a maximum but limited risk for any given person, *i.e.,* the concept that
contributing factors are cumulative only to a specific upper limit." This is, of
course, pure speculation and thus far is not backed by any experimental data.

Nevertheless, the clinical and epidemiologic significance of these observations
is clear. First, they provide a logical response to critics of the epidemiologic
studies who have suggested that endometrial cancer is merely unmasked earlier
in constitutionally predisposed estrogen users, by virtue of the fact that they are
relatively affluent and have easy access to medical care. If this objection were

Table 4. Parity in Postmenopausal Endometrial
Carcinoma Patients With and Without Prior Estrogen
Exposure

	No Estrogen (73)	Estrogen (38)
0	25	9
1	16	7
2	14	12
3–5	13	8
6 or more	5	2

true, it might indicate that the increased risk in estrogen users is apparent rather than real. However, studies such as the present one, which show that the commonly accepted constitutional risk factors are less common in estrogen users than nonusers with endometrial cancer, seem to discredit at least this one objection to the epidemiologic data.

The second important significance of these observations lies in the fact that the risk of development of endometrial cancer cannot be avoided simply by withholding estrogens from constitutionally predisposed women, as defined by these clinical parameters. Thus, if we accept that the risk is real, the solution must be more complicated.

Experimental data in animal systems would lead us to expect that the risk of constitutional factors and environmental ones should indeed be additive, rather than mutually exclusive, as suggested by the present study. For example, in rabbits, one of the few species to develop spontaneous endometrial carcinoma, Greene and Saxton (17) have demonstrated the presence of the common clinical markers, usually in old breeders. Burrows (18) has shown a 60% incidence of endometrial carcinoma in virginal animals, as have Hass et al. (19). In producing tumors with 2-AAF, Hass has shown a protective effect of oophorectomy in the induction of both endometrial and bladder carcinomas. Thus, the apparent differences in human data remain to be explained.

Other clinical factors evaluated included the time between the last normal menstrual period and the diagnosis of carcinoma and the duration of symptoms before diagnosis. The former of these determinations was similar for estrogen users and nonusers, the mean times being 13.6 and 12.0 years, respectively. The data for duration of symptoms revealed a somewhat more impressive disparity, with users having had the definitive diagnosis made in an average of 4.6 months from the onset of symptomatology, while nonusers were symptomatic for a mean duration of 7.8 months. Thus, these data do indeed confirm the suggestion that estrogen users are either more likely to report symptoms earlier or tend to receive better medical care in terms of early evaluation of these symptoms. In all patients, as expected, by far the most common symptom was postmenopausal vaginal bleeding.

Despite the earlier diagnosis in estrogen users, however, there was little evidence of differences in extent of disease between the two groups. Table 5 shows the retrospective clinical staging, as obtained from data in the clinical charts. Information was inadequate for accurate clinical staging in several patients in

Table 5. Retrospective Clinical Staging in Estrogen Users and Nonusers

FIGO Stage	No Estrogen	Estrogen
I	50	21
II	10	6
III	2	0
IV	2	2
Unknown	11	10

each group, but of the remainder there was an overwhelming tendency to "early" disease, as defined by FIGO clinical stages I and II, in both estrogen users and nonusers, with the vast majority of patients in both groups being placed in stage I.

Within clinical stage I, however, there was a greater tendency toward stage IA among estrogen users than nonusers (12 of 16 in whom this information was available in the former group versus 22 of 40 in the latter). This tendency was confirmed by examination of microscopic slides from the hysterectomies that were performed. Twenty-three of 38 uteri with residual tumor from estrogen nonusers demonstrated myometrial invasion, in contrast with only 11 of 29 specimens from estrogen users. However, since 14 nonuser uteri and six user uteri showed no residual tumor in the hysterectomy specimen, and because we have not yet completed our analysis of prehysterectomy therapy given to these patients, it is too early to determine the significance of these results.

Analysis of the histologic type and grade of the tumors seen in the two groups revealed one major difference (Table 6). Mixed adenosquamous carcinoma

Table 6. Histologic Type and Grade of Carcinoma in Estrogen Users and Nonusers

	No Estrogen (75)	Estrogen (39)
Adenocarcinoma	36	23
Grade I	28	19
Grade II	6	4
Grade III	2	0
Adenoacanthoma	13	8
Mixed adenosquamous	21	6
Clear cell	3	0
Secretory	1	1
Inadequate specimen	1	1

comprised 28% of cases in nonusers versus only 15% of cases in estrogen users. The former figure is very close to the figure of 32% quoted for the incidence of this tumor type in recent years by Reagan (20), while 15% appears to be an underrepresentation. Since this tumor is thought to have a particularly poor prognosis (21, 22), this is further evidence of a slightly more favorable type of disease in estrogen users. However, among the pure adenocarcinomas, which comprised the most frequent type in both groups of patients, the vast majority were well differentiated (grade I) in both users and nonusers.

Other histopathologic factors studied showed varying patterns. Vascular invasion was searched for in hysterectomy specimens with routine staining techniques only and was identified in only a small minority of cases. It was, however, several times more common among nonusers (10 of 54 cases) than users (two of 37).

On the other hand, both ciliated cells and clear cells, which are generally accepted as markers of estrogenic stimulation in benign endometria (23), were found more frequently in estrogen-related tumors. Table 7 shows the figures for clear cells, and Table 8 lists the data for ciliated cells.

Table 7.   Clear Cells in Endometrial Carcinoma

	No Estrogen	Estrogen
Absent	30	9
Few	27	23
Many	14	6
Not applicable (clear cell or secretory carcinoma)	4	1

Table 8.   Ciliated Cells in Endometrial Carcinoma

	No Estrogen	Estrogen
Absent	69	24
Rare	2	9
Prominent	4	6

The incidence of associated endometrial hyperplasia in either the curettage or hysterectomy specimen showed no significant difference between estrogen users and nonusers. Only 25% of users and 20% of nonusers failed to exhibit hyperplasia in at least one slide. Thus, there is no evidence for the assumption that the tumors in either group might have developed frequently without the intermediary hyperplastic lesion.

Similarly, there was no significant difference in the frequency of lymphocytic and plasma cell infiltrates between the tumors of estrogen users and nonusers. Moderate or marked degrees of such infiltration were seen in 31% of estrogen users and in 40% of nonusers. The infiltrates were evaluated only in nonnecrotic tumor foci and thus may provide an indication of host defense against tumor proliferation.

Although the follow-up period for these patients tends to be short, averaging only 3 years in both estrogen users and nonusers, an important difference is already discernible in tumor-free survival patterns. Of the 31 estrogen-related cases with some follow-up data available, two patients have died of intercurrent disease without evidence of recurrent cancer, and one patient is living with recurrent tumor. On the other hand, of 66 estrogen nonusers with follow-up information, seven have died of intercurrent disease or unknown cause, seven are known to be dead of endometrial cancer, and seven are living with documented tumor recurrence. Thus, even though clinical staging and histologic grading fail to reveal remarkable differences between the two groups, the differences in results of treatment are thus far striking. We cannot guarantee that more estrogen-related cases will not begin to recur and to show a lethal outcome as the follow-up period lengthens, but at least at this time the disease appears to behave in a significantly more "benign" fashion in this group of women. This is true despite the fact that some, albeit a minority, of these women do indeed have high-grade tumors and definite myometrial invasion. We are intrigued by the possibility that the removal of exogenous estrogen from the environment of these patients may limit the potential of these tumors for continued growth and metastasis. Obviously, the potential for controlled clinical trials is limited, but if these cases continue to do well, they will be an important factor in the risk/benefit evaluation of exogenous estrogens in postmenopausal women.

REFERENCES

1. Allen E: Ovarian hormones and female genital cancer. J Amer Med Ass **114**:2107, 1940.

2. Geist SH, Solmon UJ: Are estrogens carcinogenic in the human female? Amer J Obstet Gynecol **41**:39, 1941.

3. Knab DR: Estrogen and endometrial carcinoma. Obstet Gynecol Surv **32**:267, 1977.

4. Smith DC, Prentice R, Thompson DJ, et al: Association of exogenous estrogen and endometrial carcinoma. N Engl J Med **293**:1164, 1975.

5. Ziel HK, Finkle WD: Increased risk of endometrial carcinoma among users of conjugated estrogens. N Engl J Med **293**:1167, 1975.

6. Gray LA Sr, Christopherson WM, Hoover R: Estrogens and endometrial carcinoma. Obstet Gynecol **49**:385, 1977.

7. Mack TM, Pike MC, Henderson BE, et al: Estrogens and endometrial cancer in a retirement community. N Engl J Med **294**:1262, 1976.

8. McDonald TW, Annegers GF, O'Fallon WM, et al: Exogenous estrogen and endometrial carcinoma: case-control and incidence study. Amer J Obstet Gynecol **127**:572, 1977.

9. Doll R, Kinlen LJ, Skegg DCG, et al: Hormone replacement therapy and endometrial carcinoma (Letter to the Editor). Lancet **I**:745, 1977.

10. Gordon GS, Greenberg BG: Exogenous estrogens and endometrial cancer. Postgrad Med **59**:66, 1976.

11. Greenblatt RB, Bryner JR: The pill and cancer: was the judgment too hasty? Curr Prescribing **3**:59, 1977.

12. Weiss NS, Szekely DR, Austin DF: Increasing incidence of endometrial cancer in the United States. N Engl J Med **294**:1259, 1976.

13. Sommers SC, Hertig AT, Bengloff H: Genesis of endometrial carcinoma. II. Cases 19–35 years old. Cancer **2**:957, 1949.

14. Mansell H, Hertig AT: Granulosa-theca cell tumors and endometrial carcinoma. Obstet Gynecol **6**:385, 1955.

15. Dockerly MB, Mussey E: Malignant lesions of the uterus associated with estrogen producing ovarian tumors. Amer J Obstet Gynecol **64**:147, 1954.

16. Gompel C, Silverberg SG: *Pathology in Gynecology and Obstetrics*. Philadelphia, JB Lippincott, 1977, 2nd edit, p. 204.

17. Greene HSN, Saxton JA Jr: Uterine adenomata in the rabbit. I. Clinical history, pathology, and preliminary transplantation experiments. J Exp Med **67**:691, 1938.

18. Burrows H: Spontaneous uterine and mammary tumors in rabbit. J Pathol Bacteriol **51**:385, 1940.

19. Hass GM, et al: Personal communication.

20. Reagan JW: The changing nature of endometrial cancer. Gynecol Oncol **2**:144, 1974.

21. Ng ABP, Reagan JW, Storaasli JP, et al: Mixed adenosquamous carcinoma of the endometrium. Amer J Clin Pathol **59**:765, 1973.

22. Silverberg SG, Bolin MG, DeGiorgi LS: Adenoacanthoma and mixed adenosquamous carcinoma of the endometrium. A clinicopathologic study. Cancer **30**:1307, 1972.

23. Silverberg SG: *Surgical Pathology of the Uterus*. New York, John Wiley & Sons, 1977, pp. 17,33.

Postmenopausal Estrogens and Endometrial Cancer: A Pathologist's Overview

Sheldon C. Sommers, M.D.

No known natural hormone has been proved to be a cause of any human cancer.

When the increase in endometrial carcinoma incidence at a rate changing from 15 to 26/100,000 women per year (1) is linked to use of postmenopausal estrogen, the onus is placed on the agents, whereas it is equally likely that a karyotypically abnormal subgroup destined to develop endometrial carcinoma anyway is being identified. Until sufficient chromosomal studies are made of women with endometrial carcinoma and their relatives, there is no certainty as to whether the host or the environment is to be considered basically most at fault. It has been said that we fear to examine ourselves and prefer to blame the environment for disease.

Cause needs defining, and for scientific purposes, a causative agent must be both necessary and sufficient. Are unopposed estrogens necessary for the development of human endometrial carcinoma? Not always, evidently, since virilized women (2), individuals with Turner's ovarian aplasia (3), and women postoophorectomy (4) occasionally develop this tumor. Estrogens are, however, usually necessary as a permissive factor. This means that estrogens form a part of the endocrine environment in which endometrial carcinoma ordinarily develops.

Are estrogens sufficient by themselves to induce endometrial carcinoma? Both experimentally and clinicopathologically, clearly no. Estrogens are not cell transformers, which means that they do not stimulate an alteration in nuclear DNA that irreversibly changes cells into the neoplastic state (5, 6). Estrogens are growth stimulants, not cancer initiators. This is not a trivial or academic distinction. It is a basic fact of both theoretical and practical importance. Growth stimulants are legion and include insulin, growth hormone, amino acids, polypeptides and proteins (7, 8).

Skin, because of its accessibility, constitutes the tissue where experimental carcinogenesis is currently in the most advanced state of knowledge. Boutwell (9) has developed a scheme of interrelating the steps in skin carcinogenesis that involve neoplastic cellular transformation and subsequent stimulation to cancer outgrowth (Figure 1). Note that hormonal effects occur near the end of the multistage process, as growth stimulants, not initiators.

Once estrogens are recognized as growth stimulants, their participation in the cellular and tissue alterations that culminate in cancer can be dealt with rationally. One accepts that skin and endometrium are different, that radioimmunoassays of blood estrogens and estrogen receptor studies have not been performed in enough individuals to provide a complete and satisfying picture, and that more is unknown than known about endometrial carcinogenesis. Yet, the distinction between carcinogens and growth stimulants remains crucial.

Politicizers, writers who emphasize medical bad news, and professional consumer advocates usually blur or deny these important distinctions, either through ignorance or venally. Thus, at the Federal Drug Administration hearing on conjugated estrogens, the author understood a speaker to say that drug companies were making millions killing women with endometrial cancer.

An FDA Director (10) considered that statements by individual physicians who had not observed an increase in incidence of endometrial cancer in their patients taking estrogens can by no means be responsibly designated as evidence. Statistics is evidently the only true governmental religion.

Sometimes a growth stimulant is stigmatized as a cocarcinogen. This term is correctly defined as "a substance that promotes the development of cancer in the presence of a carcinogen." For the endometrium, the only carcinogenic agent so far known is ionizing radiation (11). In Japanese atomic bomb survivors, no statistically significant increase in endometrial carcinoma has been reported (12).

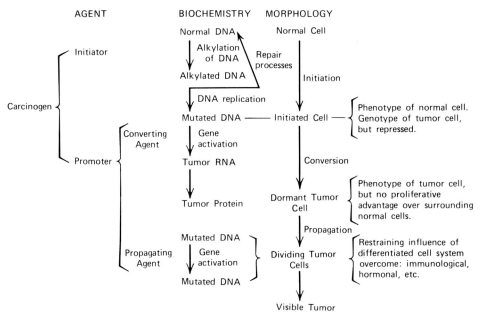

Figure 1. A schematic summary of two-stage carcinogenesis showing the biochemical changes associated with each agent and the cell state. A promoter is shown as having two attributes, conversion and propagation, both based on the property of gene activation. [Reprinted with permission from RK Boutwell: The function and mechanism of promoters of carcinogenesis. CRC Crit Rev Toxicol **2**:419, 1974. Copyright The Chemical Rubber Co CRC Press, Inc.]

Hence, it may be concluded that radiation is not carcinogenic in women with cyclic menstrual endometria. For them, irradiation is not significantly carcinogenic; therefore, cyclic estrogens cannot be cocarcinogenic.

However, ionizing radiation is carcinogenic for noncyclic proliferative endometrium with endometrial hyperplasia (11, 13). Here is a general oncologic principle with a specific application to endometrium: tissues with increased proliferation (mitoses, DNA turnover) are at increased risk of radiation carcinogenesis. The thyroid gland is an example, in that irradiation damage is much more carcinogenic before age 20 years than afterward, because thyroid mitoses and cell turnover rates are greatly reduced in adults (14).

Normally, from the menarche until the age of about 40–45 years, the endometrium is deciduous. It is cast off monthly, and no tissue substrate persists to develop hyperplasia, dysplasia, or cancer. At risk are women who have a persisting endometrium that proliferates, that is, those with many consecutive anovulatory cycles. After four or more sequential anovulatory cycles, proliferative endometrium develops into cystic glandular hyperplasia. After six or more such consecutive cycles, outpouched endometrial glands with adenomatous hyperplasia may develop. After more months or years of uninterrupted endometrial growth, that is, in the presence of no postovulatory menstruation and no pregnancy, endometrial atypia or dysplasia may develop (15). A thorough curettage that removes this hyperplastic overgrowth of endometrium is sufficient therapy, not followed by a regrowth of hyperplasia in about 75% of women (16).

So far as is known, continuous endogenous estrogenic stimulation will lead to cystic hyperplasia, adenomatous hyperplasia, and dysplasia of the endometrium. Endometrium will respond to estrogenic stimulation to this extent and no further. Note that cystic hyperplasia involves an even epithelial rate of growth all along the gland lining, and the result is a uniform spherical expansion. One might call this "Boyle's law of the endometrium." However, in adenomatous hyperplasia and dysplasia, there is an irregular growth, with a budding outward of the more active cells. Target organ sensitivity to growth stimulation in the latter lesions varies from cell to cell and from gland to gland.

Because there is as yet no way to measure differences in individual target cell responsiveness, we tend to ignore what is probably the most crucial issue in endocrine carcinogenesis, namely, irregular local target organ reactivity. In endometrium, breast, prostate, thyroid, adrenal cortex, and elsewhere, the whole tissue may not respond evenly. Carcinomas develop locally, the *raison d'être* of surgical therapy.

Putting these two facts together, continued endometrial growth and localized target organ overreaction, let us examine the youngest women with endometrial carcinoma. Most of those aged 35 years or less have polycystic ovaries or ovarian thecomatosis (17). Such ovaries secrete estrogens continuously, as well as partial or complete androgens, but no progestogens. This situation provides an unremitting stimulus for endometrial growth, because ovulation rarely, if ever, occurs, and, consequently, pregnancy is virtually impossible. The endometrium is neither cast off by menstruation nor converted to decidua of pregnancy with arrested glandular growth for 9 months.

Also, about 50% of such women are karyotypically abnormal, usually with chromosomal mosaicism of XX/XO, XX/XXY, and so on (18–20). They have indeed a form of gonadal dysgenesis, sometimes with virilizing sex cord cells in the ovary (21). Why is this important? It is because individuals with gonadal chromosomal abnormalities are prone to have nuclear DNA instability and to develop chromosomal alterations that predispose to cancers of the gonads and their target organs. Klinefelter's syndrome (XXY) is another example of gonadal dysgenesis in which an enhanced tendency to malignant cell transformation is known clinically and demonstrable experimentally (22, 23).

Here are two pieces of the puzzle fitted together: genetically unstable nuclei and continuous growth stimulation. What is the relevance to endometrial cancer in general? First, it is that the original cancer family G of Warthin and other comparable families followed by Lynch and Krush (24) have a tendency to endometrial carcinoma and to gastrointestinal carcinomas in both sexes. The familial endometrial carcinoma syndrome, which displays a dominant inheritance, accounts for about 13% of the cases collected by Lynch (22). Another similar family recently reported had both a chromosomal abnormality and T-cell immunodeficiency, encouraging the outgrowth of cancers (25, 26). A minority, to be sure, but an instructive one, because a genotype for endometrial carcinoma is now established.

There is an abnormal female somatotype found in about 30–50% of endometrial carcinoma patients. It is the "burgeoning woman" of Corscaden, who is big boned, obese, and has a tendency to reduced glucose tolerance or diabetes mellitus, hypertension, and degenerative arthritis (27). These body changes and metabolic abnormalities represent consequences of anterior pituitary hyperfunction, especially of increased growth hormone, ACTH, and gonadotropins. The metabolic abnormalities share some features of Cushing's syndrome (hypercortisolism). Familial cases have this phenotype in some instances.

Do burgeoning women have a karyotypic abnormality, such as gonadal or endometrial mosaicism? This possibility has not been specifically studied and is not known. In familial endometrial carcinoma cases, the implication is that they do.

This brings us to consideration of the great majority of women with endometrial carcinoma, of average age 57–58 years, and a majority in the age range of 45–70 years. They have a tendency to be of upper economic classes, to marry late or remain single, to be sterile or to have had few pregnancies, and to be overweight. Most are white.

Their endometrium appears to have been normal 12 or more years before carcinoma was diagnosed. Within the 10-year period before cancer was found, they had cystic hyperplasia, adenomatous hyperplasia, dysplasia, and perhaps endometrial carcinoma in situ at progressively shorter intervals antedating cancer (28, 29). Hyperplasia probably represents the usual precursor of endometrial carcinoma (30). Sufficient precancerous endometrial biopsies are not available, but it appears that all cases do not pass sequentially through all types of hyperplasia.

The hyperplastic way stations on the route to endometrial carcinoma are as far as most women go. Only about 12–15% of women with adenomatous endometrial hyperplasia and dysplasia proceed to develop endometrial carcinoma; more than 80% do not (31). Of course, there is a fundamental problem here, because it is impossible both to remove endometrium for diagnosis and to leave it to grow undisturbed. Recall that after a single curettage, about 75% of women have no recurrence of hyperplasia.

From what is known, only a small minority of women with endometrial hyperplasia progress to the development of endometrial carcinoma. In those with carcinoma in situ, the average age is 48–49, as compared to average age of 57–58 years for invasive endometrial carcinoma (32). What distinguishes this subgroup? We do not know for certain, but they appear to have a greater focal endometrial epithelial instability, perhaps both inherited and chromosomal, and a greater tendency toward malignant endometrial cell transformation after ir-radiation or other stimuli (?oncogenes, ?viruses).

Based on evidence from experimental endometrial carcinogenesis in rabbits and other investigations, estrogenic growth stimulation only results in priming the endometrium to become hyperplastic, because after estrogen withdrawal or curettage, the hyperplasia reverts to atrophy. This hyperplasia is the first stage of endometrial cancer development. In this first stage, progestagen administration also results in the reversion of hyperplasia to atrophy. The endometrium retains its usual hormonal dependency (33–35).

The second stage of carcinogenesis is different, and estrogens evidently are not essential. Morphologically, the changes are endometrial carcinoma in situ, early invasive and overtly invasive carcinoma. This chapter is not an exercise to teach diagnostic criteria, which are given elsewhere. However, an accurate endometrial diagnosis requires some skill and experience, which are not au-tomatically conferred by Board certification. Mistaking chronic endometritis, squamous metaplasia, secretory exhaustion, pseudodecidua, and cytologic and glandular atypia for carcinoma simply leads to confusion.

The second stage of endometrial carcinogenesis involves both a host endocrine and tissue overreaction. In rabbits and some women, a constellation of anterior pituitary and adrenocortical hyperfunction with morphologic hyperplasias is involved, perhaps secondary to hypothalamic dysfunction (36, 37). These findings may be epiphenomena, not nearly so critical as neoplastic endometrial cell transformation, which present techniques do not identify, except for nuclear aneuploidy (30). The adrenocortical hypersecretion of androstenedione and its peripheral transformation into estrone, particularly notable in obese women, may be important (38). This is because estrogens are hormones with different dose levels of effect, since small amounts stimulate and large amounts inhibit tissue growth. Here, this author speculates why obesity and thus larger amounts of estrone converted from androstenedione are meaningful. It is because once endometrial hyperplasia has developed, hormonal inhibition of cell growth may encourage neoplastic transformation. This situation is believed to occur in pros-tatic carcinogenesis, where carcinoma arises in foci of glandular atrophy, not hyperplasia, consequent to hormonal stimulation and its sequelae (39).

Endometrial carcinoma in situ is the only noninvasive carcinoma characterized by hypochromatic (not hyperchromatic) nuclei (15). What this hypochromatism means is unknown. Perhaps it may indicate a temporary loss of estrogen and progestagen receptors and a consequent temporary release from hormonal con-trol of endometrial cell and tissue growth.

To summarize again the events in endometrial carcinogenesis: a woman who may have a chromosomal instability of the gonadal and endometrial cells passes through an approximately 10-year period of anovulatory cycles with continuous endometrial growth, stimulated by estrogens. For genetic or unknown reasons, this first stage of endometrial hyperplasia is succeeded by a second stage of hypothalamic-pituitary-adrenocortical hyperfunction that accompanies or encourages carcinomatous endometrial transformation and outgrowth of a carcinoma that is recognizable clinically and pathologically.

During this two-stage process, the woman's blood and urinary estrogen levels are increased significantly above normal (40). This point is mentioned again later. Other hormones have not been so well studied, but, at least sometimes, pituitary luteinizing hormone, ACTH, growth hormone, androstenedione, and cortisol are also increased in the circulating blood. In both patients and experimental rabbits, the endometrial carcinoma develops over about one-seventh of the normal life-span (15, 33). Rabbits carefully maintained to very old age develop endometrial carcinoma without any experimental manipulation. Rabbits also have the *gs* antigen indicator of a viral oncogene (15). Depot estrogen acts to encourage the earlier development of a cancer to which the rabbit is constitutionally disposed. The predisposition involves a specific target organ susceptibility plus an inferred oncogene. The situation in mouse mammary carcinogenesis is similar.

After this rather long preamble concerning the natural history of endometrial carcinogenesis, let us consider the assigned topic, administration of estrogens to perimenopausal and postmenopausal women.

There have been scattered individual case reports for more than 30 years of endometrial carcinoma induced by estrogen administration. These reports include estrogen given to patients with gonadal dysgenesis or Turner's syndrome or after oophorectomy (41, 42). This author adds a case of a man aged 82 years treated with estrogens for prostatic carcinoma who developed endometrial carcinoma of the prostatic uterus masculinus, along with estrogenization of the utricular surface mucosa. He also had a papillary urothelial carcinoma of the bladder neck (triple primary cancers).

These case reports share the characteristics of having a prior genital tract abnormality that was recognized and treated, a rather prolonged exposure to estrogen therapy, and a rather high dose level. They demonstrate that estrogens can play a significant background role, as a growth promoter or possibly as a contributory cause of endometrial carcinoma in the predisposed individual.

The current wave of interest in estrogen administration and endometrial carcinoma derives from a series of epidemiologic studies reported in *The New England Journal of Medicine* (43–45) and the subsequent widespread media publicity, controversy, and governmental FDA intervention. The author has been interested in epidemiologic research since about 1950. The author's opinion is that statistical epidemiology is a young and desperate science, because it has no generally observed standards, rules, or quality controls and because it may lend itself to "statistical malpractice" (46). It is the author's belief that it is a soft science like sociology, economics, and psychiatry. Medawar (47) has called it an unnatural science. Graham Greene wrote that modern myths are medical. The real tragedy of late twentieth century America is that the pronouncements of epidemiologist-statisticians are seized upon uncritically by government as the basis for peremptory actions, usually prohibitory in nature. Correction of the excessive governmental controls comes slowly limping after.

Feinstein (46, 48, 49) has written extensively and elegantly on the proper and improper practice of epidemiology and statistics. Without going into a detailed, formal criticism of the statistical epidemiology of estrogen administration and endometrial cancer incidence, some simple points may be raised:

1. Statistical mathematics applies chiefly to the comparison of random groups. All of the women taking estrogens were selected by their doctors or themselves. The women using estrogen were a selected nonrandom population.

The controls may or may not have been selected. Women with cervical and ovarian cancer employed as controls in the Smith et al. study (43) have special selective characteristics, as is well known. In fact, economically, socially, reproductively, and in other ways, women with cervical carcinoma are practically the antithesis of women with endometrial carcinoma (50). Failure to correct for the rather large group of hysterectomized women clearly not at risk of developing endometrial carcinoma among the controls also has been thought to bias some studies (51).

Comparison of selected groups by a mathematics that applies only to random groups could give a valid answer only by lucky chance. Statisticians like to neglect this particularly crucial shortcoming as if it did not exist.

2. A serious defect in retrospective case control studies is the one to one comparison of experimental and control groups (smoker-nonsmoker, tuberculous-nontuberculous, estrogen-nonestrogen) under the mistaken assumption that in all other respects, the two groups are comparable. This assumption results sometimes in the Berkson fallacy, in which one subgroup is notably underrepresented, such as women who neither have had their endometrium examined nor taken estrogens.

Multifactorial statistical analyses are more likely to put so-called risk factors into proper perspective. For example, Rose and Bell (52) found that the multifactorial analysis of early deaths in men dropped cigarette smoking from the most significant, as found by a one to one comparison, to somewhere beyond the 30th most significant factor. In endometrial carcinoma, multifactorial analysis (53) has suggested that obesity is the most important related factor, followed by tallness, increased blood pressure, hyperglycemia, heavy menses, and late menopause.

3. Accurate diagnosis is crucial to any proper epidemiologic study. The overused trite analogy of the pump handle and the cholera epidemic comes off poorly if many of the victims had something else, such as diarrhea from pellagra.

In two of the studies cited (43, 44), there was no prior review of the endometrial specimens to determine if carcinoma was actually present. The diagnostic reports were blindly accepted. However, Gordon et al. (63) have admitted that all three of the experts who reviewed material from the cases of Ziel and Finkle (44) concurred in the diagnosis of carcinoma in only 74% of cases.

A 25% error in entry diagnosis may be acceptable epidemiologically, but no pathologist could hold a job with this overall rate of error. If such a low accuracy rate of pathologic diagnosis is acceptable to epidemiologist-statisticians, theirs is truly a crude and blunt scientific instrument. If the incidence rate of endometrial carcinoma rose during a period when 25% of the diagnoses were erroneous, was the increase significant? The author leaves the answer to the more mathematically gifted.

In another report (45), one third of the endometrial carcinomas were classified as noninvasive, whatever that means. Literally, noninvasive refers to carcinoma in situ, but so many were reported that either there was a gross overdiagnosis or noninvasive means something else. Perhaps it actually is intended to indicate that the myometrium was not invaded. If so, as pointed out by Kistner (5), many endometrial carcinomas were in clinical stages 0 or 1, which should not be equated with the ordinary group of women reported with clinical endometrial carcinoma.

4. No one knows the pretreatment status of the endometrium or, in the controls, the status of the endometrium at any time. If the estrogen-treated women already had or were particularly predisposed to endometrial hyperplasia, the risk factor calculations become mumbo jumbo. As has been pointed out, the indications for treatment, the treatment schedules, dosages, and data on the continuance of therapy are not given.

If women with endometrial carcinoma have previously had increased circulating estrogen levels, what would be the effect of adding prescribed estrogens? The answer is not known. This author speculates that it might increase the endometrial estrogen concentration from the stimulatory to the inhibitory level of tissue growth and cell turnover. If this changeover should occur in an endometrium that was already hyperplastic, dysplasia and neoplasia might be more likely to develop.

5. The increased frequency of diagnosis of endometrial carcinoma in recent decades and the increasing amounts of estrogen prescribed nationally are cited as suggesting a relationship (1). This is mere nonsense, because the same correlation would apply to color television sets, irradiation from which could be blamed. Lung cancer and the distribution of an English newspaper rose together. From this it might be inferred that *The New York Times* is dangerous to health (54).

Note that in Norway and Czechoslovakia, two countries where estrogens are not commonly prescribed, endometrial carcinoma also increased during the same period (55, 56). The authors wondered whether later marriages and fewer pregnancies might be involved. Further, the Third National Cancer Survey failed to show any United States increase in endometrial carcinoma.

6. Regional and secular differences cannot be ignored (57). Some gynecologists have prescribed estrogens for many years without any significant incidence of endometrial carcinoma in their patients (58, 59). The author's experience in the East and two years in California suggest that there are profound population differences. Perhaps women on the West Coast should not take perimenopausal estrogens, but this possible suggestion does not necessarily apply to the entire United States.

A study in Iowa demonstrated no implication of estrogen administration in endometrial carcinoma (60). In New York, this author estimates that about 1% of endometrial carcinoma may be related to estrogen administration. Higginson (61) has estimated a figure of 10% in a recent review.

To summarize this chapter, epidemiologic-statistical retrospective case control studies that were rather poorly planned and suffered from critical scientific deficiencies have failed to answer the questions of how often and how significantly perimenopausal estrogen administration may contribute to the development of endometrial carcinoma. The answers are not known, and prospective cohort studies are needed to avoid the acknowledged defects of case control and retrospective studies. In a small follow-up aspiration biopsy study of 25 women who had taken perimenopausal estrogens, performed with Dr. Penny Budoff (62), endometrial adenomatous hyperplasia was found in one person. This is a hint that perhaps one sixth of 4% (0.6%) of these women may be at risk for endometrial carcinoma after estrogen treatment.

To conclude, leaving aside the alarmist pseudoscientific discoveries of epidemiologist-statisticians and the governmental overreactions to alleged environmental hazards, both of which are unwholesome parts of our times, let us consider the patient and the doctor. If there is a family history of endometrial or gastrointestinal carcinoma; obesity, diabetes, and hypertension; proven endometrial hyperplasia or dysplasia; or an abnormal genotype, estrogens should probably not be given, because they might exaggerate an already abnormal situation and contribute eventually to endometrial carcinoma development.

In other women of menopausal age, based on reasonable clinical indications and apparent need, estrogens may be prescribed without fear of endometrial carcinogenesis, provided that an initial endometrial specimen does not exhibit hyperplasia or dysplasia, that the dose is in the low (growth stimulating) rather than in the high (growth inhibiting) range, and that the estrogen is not given continuously or, if it is, that progestagen is administered concomitantly about one week in every four. Furthermore, follow-up endometrial aspiration or curette biopsies are desirable to appraise the endometrial response at intervals. In short, in the use of estrogens, moderation is desirable.

REFERENCES

1. Greenwald P, Nasca PC, Caputo TA, et al. Cancer risks from estrogen intake. NY State J Med **77:**1069,1977.

2. Mahesh VB, McDonough PG, Greenblatt RB: Endocrine studies in a patient with virilism, ovarian stromal hyperplasia and endometrial carcinoma. Obstet Gynecol **30:**584, 1967.

3. Gray PH, Anderson CT, Munnell EW: Endometrial adenocarcinoma and ovarian agenesis. Obstet Gynecol **35:**513, 1970.

4. Hofmeister FG, Vondrak BF: Endometrial carcinoma in patients with bilateral oophorectomy. Amer J Obstet Gynecol **107:**1099, 1970.

5. Kistner RW: Endometrial cancer and estrogens (Editorial). Obstet Gynecol **48:**479, 1976.

6. Brennan MJ: Personal communication, 1976.

7. Gospodarowiecz D, Moran JS: Growth factors in mammalian cell culture. Annu Rev Biochem **45:**531, 1976.

8. Holley RW: Control of growth in mammalian cells in cell culture. Nature (London) **258:**487, 1975.

9. Boutwell RK: The function and mechanism of promoters of carcinogenesis. CRC Crit Rev Toxicol **2:**419, 1974.

10. Crout JR: Second opinion. Current Prescribing **2:**23, 1976.

11. Palmer JP, Spratt DW: Uterus cancer after x-ray irradiation. Amer J Obstet Gynecol **72**:497, 1956.

12. Steer A: The delayed consequences of exposure to ionizing radiation. Other tumors. Human Pathol **2**:541, 1971.

13. Speert H, Peightal TC: Malignant tumors of the uterine fundus subsequent to irradiation for benign pelvic conditions. Amer J Obstet Gynecol **57**:261, 1949.

14. Sommers SC: Effects of ionizing radiation upon endocrine glands, in *Pathology of Irradiation*, Berdjis CC (ed.), Baltimore, Williams & Wilkins, 1971, p. 411.

15. Sommers SC: Carcinoma of endometrium, in *The Uterus*, Norris HJ, Hertig AT, Abell MR (eds.), Baltimore, Williams & Wilkins, 1973, chap. 14, p. 276.

16. Hark B, Sommers SC: Endometrial curettage in diagnosis and therapy. Obstet Gynecol **21**:636, 1963.

17. Courey NG, Graham JB: Characteristics of women with uterine body cancer. NY State J Med **64**:1724, 1964.

18. Bishun NP, Morton WRM: Chromosome mosaicism in Stein-Leventhal syndrome. Brit Med J **2**:1200, 1964.

19. Lewis FJW, Mitchell JP, Foss GL: XY/XO mosaicism. Lancet **1**:221, 1963.

20. Moukhtar A, Aleem FA, Hung HC, et al: Reversible behavior of locally invasive endometrial carcinoma in a chromosomally mosaic pattern (45,X/46XrX) in a young woman treated with Clomid. Cancer **40**:2957, 1977.

21. Leon N, Sommers SC: Cells of masculinizing type in ovary of a patient with feminine phenotype. Acta Genet Stat Med **17**:345, 1967

22. Lynch HT: *Cancer Genetics*, Springfield, Ill., Charles C Thomas, 1976, p. 126.

23. Mukerjee D, Bowen J, Anderson DE: Simian papovavirus 40 transformation of cells from cancer patient with XY-XXY mosaic Klinefelter's syndrome. Cancer Res **30**:1769, 1970.

24. Lynch HT, Krush AJ: Cancer family "G" revisited: 1895–1970. Cancer **27**:1505, 1971; cf. also ref. 22, p. 355.

25. Law IP, Herberman RB, Oldham RK, et al: Familial occurrence of colon and uterine carcinoma and of lymphoproliferative malignancies. Cancer **39**:1224, 1977.

26. Law IP, Hollinshead AC, Whang-Peng J, et al: Familial occurrence of colon and uterine carcinoma and of lymphoproliferative malignancies. Cancer **39**:1229, 1977.

27. Gusberg SB, Frick HC II: Cancer of the endometrium, in *Corscaden's Gynecologic Cancer*, Baltimore, Williams & Wilkins, Baltimore, 1970, 4th edit.

28. Hertig AT, Sommers SC: Genesis of endometrial carcinoma. I. Study of prior biopsies. Cancer **2**:946, 1949.

29. Beutler HK, Dockerty MB, Randall LM: Precancerous lesions of the endometrium. Amer J Obstet Gynecol **86**:433, 1963.

30. Vellios F: Endometrial hyperplasias, precursors of endometrial carcinoma. Pathol Annu **7**:201, 1972.

31. Gusberg SB, Kaplan AL: Precursors of corpus cancer. Amer J Obstet Gynecol **87**:662, 1963.

32. Buehl IA, Vellios F, Carter JE, et al: Carcinoma in situ of the endometrium. Amer J Clin Pathol **42**:594, 1964.

33. Meissner WA, Sommers SC, Sherman G: Endometrial hyperplasia, endometrial carcinoma, and endometriosis produced experimentally by estrogen. Cancer **10**:500, 1957.

34. Kistner RW: The effects of progestational agents on hyperplasia and carcinoma in situ of the endometrium. Int J Gynaecol Obstet **8**:561, 1970.

35. Wentz WB: Treatment of persistent endometrial hyperplasia with progestins. Amer J Obstet Gynecol **96**:999, 1966.

36. Sommers SC, Meissner WA: Host relationships in experimental endometrial carcinoma. Cancer **10**:510, 1957.

37. Sommers SC, Meissner WA: Endocrine abnormalities accompanying endometrial cancer. Cancer **10**:516, 1957.

38. Siiteri PK, Schwarz BE, MacDonald PC: Estrogen receptors and the estrone hypothesis in relation to endometrial and breast cancer. Gynecol Oncol **2:**228, 1974.

39. Franks LM: Latent carcinoma of the prostate. J Pathol Bacteriol **68:**603, 1954.

40. Aleem FA, Moukhtar MA, Hung HC, et al: Plasma estrogen in patients with endometrial hyperplasia and carcinoma. Cancer **38:**2101, 1976.

41. Cutler BS, Forbes AP, Ingersoll FM, et al: Endometrial carcinoma after stilbestrol therapy in gonadal dysgenesis. N Engl J Med **287:**628, 1972.

42. Bromberg YM, Liban E, Laufer A: Early endometrial carcinoma following prolonged estrogen administration in an ovariectomized woman. Obstet Gynecol **14:**221, 1959.

43. Smith DC, Prentice R, Thompson DJ, et al: Association of exogenous estrogen and endometrial carcinoma. N Engl J Med **293:**1167, 1975.

44. Ziel HK, Finkle WD: Increased risk of endometrial carcinoma among users of conjugated estrogen. N Engl J Med **293:**1167, 1975.

45. Mack TE, Pike MC, Henderson BE, et al: Estrogens and endometrial cancer in a retirement community. N Engl J Med **294:**1262, 1976.

46. Feinstein AR: VI. Statistical "malpractice" and the responsibility of a consultant. Clin Pharmacol Ther **11:**898, 1970.

47. Medawar P: Unnatural science. New York Review, Feb. 3, 1977, p. 13.

48. Feinstein AR: XX. The epidemiologic trohoc, the ablative risk ratio, and retrospective research. Clin Pharmacol Ther **14:**291, 1973.

49. Horwitz RI, Feinstein AR: Post trohoc ergo propter trohoc: problems, conflicting results, and criteria for scientific standards in retrospective "case-control" research. Clin Res **24:**248A, 1976.

50. Hopps HC: Geographic pathology, in *Pathology*, Anderson WAD, Kissane JM (eds.), St. Louis, C.V. Mosby, 1977, p. 730.

51. Editor's note. Lancet **1:**746, 1977.

52. Rose CL, Bell B: *Predicting Longevity*. Lexington, Mass., Heath Lexington Books, 1971; cf. pp. xv, 128, 131, and Table 7-4.

53. Wynder EL, Escher GC, Mantel N: An epidemiological investigation of cancer of the endometrium. Cancer **19:**489, 1966.

54. Lasagna L: Unfit to print? Sciences **17:**33, 1977.

55. Setekleiv J, Borchgerink CF: Kan langvarig østrogenbehandling fremkalle livmorkreft hos postklimakteriske kvinner? Nor Laegertidj **594,** 1976.

56. Rosol M, Strnad L, Havel V, et al: Untersuchungen zum Inzidenzanstieg der Endometrium-und Ovarialkarzinome in der CSSr Während der Jahre 1960 bis 1973. Zentr Gynäkol **3:**175, 1976.

57. Rutledge FN: Estrogen therapy: a causal role in endometrial cancer? Amer J Roentgenol Radium Ther Nucl Med **127:**897, 1976.

58. Greenblatt R: Quoted by Peck RL: The estrogen-cancer flap: what you need to know. Curr Prescribing **5:**19, 1976.

59. Record JW: Endometrial cancer and estrogens. South Med J **70:**1, 1977.

60. Dunn LJ, Bradbury JT: Endocrine factors in endometrial carcinoma. Amer J Obstet Gynecol **97:**465, 1967.

61. Higginson J: The role of the pathologist in environmental medicine and public health. Amer J Pathol **86:**460, 1977.

62. Budoff PW, Sommers SC: Estrogen-progesterone therapy in perimenopausal women. Submitted for publication.

63. Gordon J, Reagan JW, Finkle WD, et al: Estrogen and endometrial carcinoma. N Engl J Med **297:**570, 1977.

Breast Cancer and Menopausal Estrogens

Ronald Ross, M.D.

Thomas Mack, M.D.

Veeba Gerkins, M.P.H.

Annlia Hill, Ph.D.

Unlike the situation with endometrial cancer, in which an association with menopausal estrogens seems clear-cut (1, 2), the problem with breast cancer remains unresolved, despite a mass of evidence implicating estrogens in mammary cancer in animal models (3–5).

We will first provide a brief discussion of exogenous menopausal estrogens and explain why their possible association with breast cancer has generated so much recent interest among epidemiologists, then review past studies and problems, and conclude by describing briefly a case-control study our group is currently conducting in an affluent retirement community south of Los Angeles.

In 1926, Loewe and Lange first demonstrated a female sex hormone in women's urine that varied with the stage of the menstrual cycle. The hormone estrogen was soon isolated and its chemical structure elucidated (6). The estrogens most commonly used for therapy in menopause are conjugated estrogens derived from pregnant mares' urine. These compounds are salts of estrogen esters that contain 50–60% sodium estrone sulfate and 20–35% sodium equilin sulfate. Their acceptance and popularity are due largely to the fact that they are less active than most available preparations in recommended dosages, are relatively inexpensive, and are effective orally (6).

There are two major reasons why we are interested in exogenous menopausal estrogen use and breast cancer. First, and most importantly, it makes sense that estrogens should be involved in breast cancer development. Evidence for a role of estrogens comes from four main sources:

1. Breast cancer is a hormonal cancer, which means that it arises from tissues normally responsive to endogenous hormones and that its course can be

This study was supported by Contract NO-CP-53500, Grant PO ICA 17054-01, and Grant CA 14089-03 from the National Cancer Institute.

55

influenced, either favorably or unfavorably, by administration of hormones or by hormonal manipulation (7). Various breast cancer risk factors, particularly those related to menstrual and reproductive events, support a hormonal basis for breast cancer (Table 1). For example, early age at menarche, late age at

Table 1. Known Risk Factors in Female Breast Cancer [From Henderson et al. (32). By permission of Academic Press.]

Demographic	Old age
	High socioeconomic status
	Caucasian
Menstrual	Early age at menarche
	Late age at menopause
	Decreased frequency of artificial menopause
Reproductive	Never married
	Late age at first full-term delivery
	Low parity
Other	History of benign breast disease
	Family history of breast cancer
	Increased total body size
Hormonal	Increased use of exogenous estrogens (?)

menopause (natural or artificial), late age at first full-term pregnancy, and low parity are all breast cancer risk factors, and all focus attention on the endocrine system, particularly the pituitary-gonadal axis. It seems likely that other important breast cancer risk factors, such as social class and race (9), may be related to menstrual and reproductive factors, particularly age at first pregnancy (e.g., higher-class women presumably marry later and have a later first pregnancy). Recent studies have suggested that the increased risk conveyed by a family history of breast cancer may also depend on these endocrine-related events; that is, first-degree relatives of breast cancer patients tend to have early menarche, late first full-term pregnancy, and few total pregnancies, just like the cases themselves (10).

2. Animal studies have not dampened the concept of a hormonal basis of breast cancer. The original estrogen studies in animals were performed in the late 1930s by Lipschutz and Varga (11) and Lacassagne (12), who showed a high incidence of malignant mammary tumors in highly inbred tumor-prone mice given large doses of estrogens. Since that time, increases in the amount of several circulating hormones, including the estrogen fractions estrone and estradiol [the two major fractions with growth-promoting potential in man (13)], as well as progesterone and prolactin, whether given by injection, implantation, or interference in normal feedback mechanisms (14, 15), have been shown to increase the frequency of mammary cancer in mice. Ovariectomy, on the other hand, has been shown to have a protective effect (16). It is now known that estrogens can, in fact, produce tumors regularly in a wide variety of organs, including the cervix, endometrium, ovary, and mammary gland, in a large variety of animal species, such as dogs, cats, mice, rats, and guinea pigs (17).

3. In addition to the indirect evidence suggested by the known breast cancer risk factors, there is more direct human evidence for the role of estrogens in breast cancer etiology. These studies, which have looked directly at hormonal levels, have been of two main types: studies of individuals and correlative studies of populations. Results of the former, most of which have looked at hormonal levels in the urine of breast cancer cases and controls, have generally been disappointing. Urinary levels of estrone and estradiol have been found to be elevated, similar, or even decreased compared to controls in various populations (18–20). However, more recently and more encouragingly, breast cancer patients have been demonstrated to have higher plasma estradiol levels than controls (21).

Realizing that the hormonal pattern present at the time of disease may not reflect the pattern responsible for the disease and that the disease itself may alter hormonal levels, our group has measured hormonal levels in teenage daughters of breast cancer cases (high risk) compared to control daughters (low risk). The former had significantly higher levels of luteal-phase total estrogen, progesterone, and prolactin and high but not significant elevations of follicular-phase total estrogen (10). When this study was expanded to include daughters of cases with bilateral breast cancer, an even higher-risk group, the differences for many hormones were even larger (Table 2) (22).

Table 2. Geometric Mean Plasma Levels of Various Hormones in Daughters of Women With Bilateral Breast Cancer Compared to Controls [From Henderson et al. (22).]

Hormone	Day of Menstrual Cycle	Bilateral Breast Cancer Daughters	Number Sampled	Percentage Difference From Controls
Estrone (E_1)	11	5.7	18	43[a]
Estradiol (E_2)	11	7.2	18	22
$E_1 + E_2$	11	13.1	18	31
Estrone	22	8.9	18	41
Estradiol	22	12.1	18	20
$E_1 + E_2$	22	21.3	18	27
Progesterone	22	371.3	11	26
FSH	11	10.0	18	32[a]
Prolactin	11	20.0	11	11
Prolactin	22	17.7	11	−5

[a] $p < 0.05$ by Mann-Whitney U test.

International studies have also focused on high- and low-risk breast cancer populations. Specifically, it has been shown that high-risk American Caucasian women have a lower urinary estriol ratio (estriol/estrone plus estradiol) than do low-risk Asian women, while Asian women in Hawaii, an intermediate-risk group, also have an intermediate ratio (23). The estriol ratio hypothesis has developed because estriol is thought to act physiologically as an antiestrogen because of its ability to compete with estradiol for estrogen-binding sites (13). However, the lower estriol ratios in the Caucasian group in this series resulted largely from 75% increases in mean urinary estrone and estradiol, since estriol levels were quite similar to those in Asian women. Therefore, the importance of this hypothesis in explaining international breast cancer rates is unclear.

4. Perhaps the most important piece of evidence, however, comes from previous studies that demonstrated that various types of exogenous estrogens can cause tumors in man: adenocarcinoma of the vagina in women exposed to the synthetic, nonsteroidal estrogen diethylstilbestrol (DES) in utero (24), liver adenoma in long-term users of oral contraceptives (25), and endometrial cancer in users of menopausal estrogens (1, 2).

In addition to the biologic plausibility for a role of estrogens in breast cancer, the interest in estrogens has increased in the past decade due to the high frequency of both exposure and disease. Premarin alone is currently the fifth most frequently prescribed drug in the country, with more than five million prescriptions annually, dollar sales having more than quadrupled since 1960 (Table 3) (26). There is also evidence that breast cancer rates have been rising during the past decade (27).

Table 3. Estimated Number (in thousands) of Annual New Estrogen Prescriptions, 1963–75 (Courtesy of IMS America Ltd., July 1975)

Year	All Estrogens	Percentage Increase Over 1963 Value	Most Popular Conjugated Estrogen Preparation	Percentage Increase Over 1963 Value
1963	2951	—	1542	—
1964	3092	5	1738	12
1965	3962	34	2432	58
1966	4902	66	3261	111
1967	5157	75	3226	109
1968	5457	85	3417	122
1969	5336	81	3446	123
1970	5968	102	3411	121
1971	6910	134	4187	172
1972	7374	150	4587	197
1973	7428	152	4780	210
1974	7741	162	4987	223

Despite the strong evidence suggesting a role for estrogens in the development of breast cancer, most studies in the literature reporting on menopausal estrogen use in breast cancer series have actually found a protective effect of these drugs. Wynder and Schneiderman summarized these studies in an editorial in the *Journal of the National Cancer Institute* in 1972, part of which has been reproduced in Table 4 (28). We suggest that all of these studies must be interpreted with

Table 4. Incidence of Breast and Gynecologic Cancer After Long-term Administration of Estrogens [From Wynder and Schneiderman (28). By permission of *Journal of the National Cancer Institute.*]

| | Number of Patients | Age (yr) | | Cancer Incidence | | |
| | | Range | Mean | Site | Observed/ Expected | Follow-up (yr) |
Authors (yr)						
Geist et al. (1941)	206	25–80		Breast and gynecologic	0/12	1–5
Henneman et al. (1957)	292	15–83	51	Gynecologic	7/22	1–25
Mustacchi & Gordon (1958)	120	15–84	62	Breast and gynecologic	0/5–6[a]	>1
Wilson (1962)	304	40–70	51	Breast and gynecologic	0/18	1–27
Schleyer-Saunders (1960)	300	30–60		Breast and gynecologic	7/Unknown	Several
Leis (1966)	158	36–54	46	Breast and gynecologic	0/Unknown	8–14
Burch & Byrd (1971)	511	27–72	54	Breast	9/39[a]	29

[a]Expected number for all malignant tumors.

caution for several reasons. First and foremost, nearly all of these studies have looked at other gynecologic cancers as well as breast cancer and have found a marked deficit in these cancers also. This finding is disturbing in view of what we now know about endometrial cancer and estrogen use (1, 2, 26). This factor, together with a deficit in general mortality in the studies that reported all deaths, suggests that incompleteness of follow-up rather than lowered risk was responsible for these results. Second, all of these studies were uncontrolled, and expected numbers were calculated from general population rates; however, it is unclear whether any of the patient series is representative of the general population in terms of breast cancer risk. Finally, the duration of follow-up in most studies was short, other breast cancer risk factors were not considered, and none examined systematically such important interacting variables as dose, duration, and method of administration.

The importance of considering other risk factors is apparent from two case-control studies our group has conducted (Table 5). These two breast cancer

Table 5. Risk of Breast Cancer in Ever Users of Menopausal Estrogens

	Patients[a]	Controls[a]	Risk Ratio
Study 1[b]	34/60	39/53	0.47
Study 2[c]	25/33	16/27	2.15
Studies 1 and 2			1.20[d]

[a] Estrogen users/total women at risk.

[b] Cases aged 50–64 matched to controls from outpatient files of same physician by race, date of birth (± 5 years), and social class.

[c] Cases aged 50–59 matched with controls by nearest-neighbor method.

[d] Estimated summary risk ratio after pooling studies and adjusting for age at diagnosis and menopause.

series yielded dramatically different results, in that the first series revealed a large protective effect for breast cancer in hormone users (8), while the second study showed a twofold increased risk (29). Estrogen use in these series was related to calendar year of diagnosis, age, and age at menopause, with the latter two factors also related to breast cancer risk. In fact, the breast cancer cases in the first series were considerably older at menopause than were the controls, which made them less likely to have used estrogens, but at increased risk for breast cancer; therefore, any increased risk related to drug use may have been masked. When we combined the studies and adjusted as best we could, we found no effect.

A study recently reported by Hoover et al. on 1891 women using conjugated estrogens for menopause and followed for an average of 12 years indicated some excess risk of developing breast cancer compared to that of the general population (30). Although the overall relative risk of 1.3 was not extraordinary (49 observed compared to 39 expected, based on general population rates), there was a suggestion that risk increased with increased follow-up and higher dose, as might be expected in a cause and effect association. The highest observed relative risk (RR) in this study was for women followed for more than 10 years who took at least 0.625 mg on other than a daily basis; RR = 4.7, with 7 observed versus 1.5 expected. This 10-year follow-up period is relevant, in that other endocrine events, such as oophorectomy, require over 10 years to show an effect on breast cancer rates (20).

In addition to the technical problems of studying this relationship that have been discussed above, two other major difficulties exist that have not yet been mentioned. First, there is a problem with respect to the latent period; that is, the critical period when we might begin to see the effect of these drugs on breast cancer rates may not yet have been reached. Although estrogens have been available for nearly 50 years (6), menopausal estrogens gained widespread acceptance only in the early 1960s (Table 3). This fact is significant since exposure to other environmental agents that act as initiators or promoters of carcinogenesis may be followed by a latent period in excess of 20 years (31). Second, it seems likely that the overall risk associated with use of exogenous estrogens will not approach the magnitude of that observed with endometrial cancer. This factor will, of course, increase the importance of identifying the inevitable low order-of-magnitude confounding factors, which will pose alternative explanations for any association to be found.

Despite these considerations, the importance of continued monitoring of this potential problem seems clear, considering the high incidence of breast cancer in the United States and the current high prevalence of exogenous estrogen use. Therefore, we have recently begun a case-control study in two retirement communities in the Los Angeles area. The primary study population is a community of 20,000 almost uniformly white, affluent persons, in whom we have been monitoring cancer incidence since 1971. The mean age of the population is about 71 years, and females outnumber males in a ratio of 5:3. Administration officials estimate that about 85% of residents attend a single medical facility and that most residents use the single pharmacy outlet within this medical facility. The second community is smaller, with just 10,000 residents, but is similar in terms of age, sex, social class, and racial composition. Again, most residents utilize the medical and pharmaceutical facilities within the community.

Breast cancer cases in these communities have been ascertained by routine surveillance of pathology records of all local hospitals, and additional cases have been detected by surveillance of all Los Angeles County hospitals by our comprehensive Cancer Surveillance Program (CSP) and from death certificates provided by local health departments. We chose to limit our study to women under 75 years of age at diagnosis, because we felt that this group would be more likely to include long-term drug users who had been taking the drugs since the onset of menopause. Furthermore, a previous study of breast cancer and reserpine use conducted in this community had included medical record abstraction of conjugated estrogen use (32) and had suggested that any excess risk might be confined to this age group (Table 6). A total of 145 individuals who satisfied this requirement and were currently alive and living in the community became the study group. Each case was matched with two controls, each drawn systematically from

Table 6. Premarin Use Ever by Age at Diagnosis[a]

Age (yr)	Fco[b]	Risk Ratio	95% Confidence Interval
< 70(39)[c]	0.22	3.1	1.40–6.01
70+(72)	0.28	1.0	0.57–1.78

[a] Data abstracted as part of a study by Mack TM, et al. (33). Cases individually matched with four community controls on date of birth and date of entry into community.

[b] Frequency of use in controls.

[c] Number of cases.

Study Population

Two retirement communities with 30,000 total population. Residents predominantly white, upper social class, elderly. Majority use single medical facility and pharmacy at each community.
Female:male ratio of 5:3

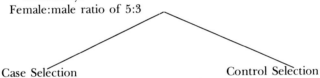

Case Selection

Routine surveillance of pathology records of all local hospitals, all Los Angeles County hospitals, and larger hospitals in surrounding counties.
Exclusions: Diagnosis before 1971
Prior breast cancer (pre-1971)
Move out
Dead
Over age 75 at diagnosis

Control Selection

Selected in a systematic fashion from a roster of community residents, matched to cases on date of birth (± 1 year), race, community entry date (± 1 year), and marital status.
Exclusions: Prior breast cancer (pre-1971)
Move out
Dead

Sources of Drug Data

Personal interview
Medical record abstraction
Pharmacy records

Figure 1. A summary of study design for detecting association between menopausal estrogen use and breast cancer in two Los Angeles retirement communities.

a complete roster of community residents. Matching was by age (± 1 year), entry date (± 1 year), marital status (ever or never married), and race. Since the community is of uniform high social class, matching was accomplished on this variable as well.

Drug histories on cases and controls are being obtained from three sources: personal interview by a trained nurse-epidemiologist, medical record abstraction by a physician-epidemiologist, and pharmacy records of estrogen prescriptions filled from 1965 to 1975 at the medical facility pharmacy. Records from the latter source will be available only from the larger community. We have not found it feasible to blind interviewers or abstractors as to case or control status. However, information on hormone use that is first noted in the medical records during the 4-month interval preceding diagnosis will be carefully excluded, thereby minimizing bias due to records present because of breast cancer symptoms in the cases. The basic design for the study is summarized in Figure 1.

Table 7 lists some of the reasons for selecting these communities as our study populations and why we feel this study can more readily detect an association between hormone usage and cancer development than could our previous surveys. First, because these are high-risk breast cancer communities with a high overall frequency of estrogen use, this study should be both sensitive and efficient in finding any relationship. Second, due to the important confounding of age at menopause, a detailed menstrual and reproductive history is being taken, which was lacking in past studies. Third, close matching of cases with community controls by age, marital status, and social class was readily achieved (in one previous study, matching was from the outpatient file of the same physician as the control, and in both previous studies, a 5-year leeway on date of

Table 7. Some Advantages of Los Angeles Retirement Communities in the Study of Menopausal Estrogen and Breast Cancer

High-risk communities (over age 65 breast cancer rates = $300/10^5$/year)

High frequency of estrogen use (about 50% overall based on previous surveys; 85% of total is conjugated estrogen)

Detailed history of menstrual and reproductive events, as well as other known breast cancer risk factors

Complete cancer surveillance in a closed community since 1971

Uniformly high social class community

Readily obtained age-matched community controls

Highly motivated and highly cooperative physicians, administrative officials, and community residents

Pharmacy prescription records as a third data source

birth was allowed). Fourth, refusal rates are low in the community, because residents are well educated, health conscious, and highly motivated to participate in medical research. Fifth, data on drug use are being obtained from three different sources, all providing detailed information on dose, duration, and type of use. Finally, it is possible that our previous surveys, which involved mainly patients aged 50–59, did not include age ranges at highest risk of getting breast cancer after exogenous hormone usage; therefore, this study encompasses a larger diagnostic age range.

Although the present study is certainly not without difficulties, we feel that these problems are inherent in any study of estrogen use and breast cancer (for example, latent period, probability of finding only a moderately high risk ratio, and recall of pertinent past events, particularly age at menopause). Despite these problems, continual monitoring is essential if epidemiologists are to determine whether exogenous menopausal estrogens are, in Wynder and Schneiderman's words, a "boon or bane" to women in terms of subsequent breast cancer risk.

SUMMARY

The role of exogenous menopausal estrogens in breast cancer etiology remains unresolved despite a mass of evidence from animal and human studies that implicates estrogens in breast cancer development. Previous studies on breast cancer risk in these hormone users have often suffered from methodologic errors and have yielded conflicting results. The methodology for a current case-control study designed to overcome these procedural and analytic errors is discussed.

REFERENCES

1. Smith DC, Prentice R, Thompson DJ, et al: Association of exogenous estrogen and endometrial carcinoma. N Engl J Med **293**:1164, 1975.

2. Ziel HK, Finkle WD: Increased risk of endometrial carcinoma among users of conjugated estrogens. N Engl J Med **293**:1167, 1975.

3. Cutts JH, Nobel RL: Estrone-induced mammary tumors in the rat. Cancer Res **24**:1116, 1964.

4. Dunning WF, Curtis MR, Segaloff A: Strain differences in response to estrone and the induction of mammary gland, adrenal and bladder cancer in rats. Cancer Res **13**:147, 1953.

5. Segaloff A, Mayfield WG: The synergism between radiation and estrogen in the production of mammary cancer in the rat. Cancer Res **31**:166, 1971.

6. Goodman LS, Gilman A (eds.): *The Pharmacological Basis of Therapeutics.* New York, Macmillan, 1970, p. 1538.

7. Zunoff B, Fishman J, Bradlow HL, et al: Hormone profiles in hormone-dependent cancers. Cancer Res **35**:3365, 1975.

8. Henderson BE, Powell D, Rosario I, et al: An epidemiologic study of breast cancer. J Nat Cancer Inst **53**:609, 1974.

9. Papaioannou N: Etiologic factors in cancer of the breast in humans. Surg Gynecol Obstet **138**:257, 1974.

10. Henderson BE, Gerkins V, Rosario I, et al: Elevated serum levels of estrogen and prolactin in daughters of patients with breast cancer. N Engl J Med **293**:790, 1975.

11. Lipschutz A, Varga L: Tumorigenic powers of stilbestrol and follicular hormones. Lancet 1:541, 1940.

12. Lacassagne A: Essai d'une hormone thyreotrope en vue de modifier l'appurition de l'adenocarcinome mammaire chez la souris. Comp Rend Soc Biol 130:591, 1939.

13. Siiteri PK, Schwartz BE, MacDonald PC: Estrogen receptors and the estrone hypothesis in relation to endometrial and breast cancer. Gynecol Oncol 2:228, 1974.

14. Muhlbock O, Boot LM: The mode of action of ovarian hormones in the induction of mammary cancer in mice. Biochem Pharmacol 16:627, 1967.

15. Welsch CW, Jenkins TW, Meites J: Increased incidence of mammary tumors in the female rat grafted with multiple pituitaries. Cancer Res 30:1024, 1970.

16. Segaloff A: The role of the ovary in estrogen production in mammary cancer in the rat. Cancer Res 34:2708, 1974.

17. Hertz R: The estrogen-cancer hypothesis. Cancer Suppl 38:534, 1976.

18. Smith WO, Emerson J: Urinary estrogens and related compounds in postmenopausal women with mammary cancers: effect of cortisone treatment. Proc Soc Exp Biol Med 85:264, 1954.

19. Breuer H, Nocke W: Chemical determination of oestrogens in the urine of women with cancer of the breast. Acta Endocrinol Suppl 31:319, 1957.

20. MacMahon B, Cole P, Brown J: Etiology of human breast cancer: a review. J Nat Cancer Inst 50:21, 1973.

21. England PL, Skinner LG, Cottrell KM, et al: Serum estradiol-17 in women with benign and malignant breast disease. Brit J Cancer 30:571, 1974.

22. Henderson BE, Pike MC, Gerkins VR, et al: The hormonal basis of breast cancer: elevated plasma levels of estrogen, prolactin and progesterone. Paper presented at the meeting Origins of Human Cancer, Cold Spring Harbor, New York, 1976.

23. MacMahon B, Cole P, Brown JB, et al: Oestrogen profiles of Asian and North American women. Lancet 2:900, 1971.

24. Herbst AL, Ulfelder H, Paskanzer DC: Adenocarcinoma of the vagina. N Engl J Med 284:878, 1971.

25. Edmondson HA, Henderson B, Benton B: Liver-cell adenomas associated with use of oral contraceptives. N Engl J Med 294:470, 1976.

26. Mack TM, Pike MC, Henderson BE, et al: Estrogens and endometrial cancer in a retirement community. N Engl J Med 294:1262, 1976.

27. Cutler SJ, Connelly RR: Mammary cancer trends. Cancer 23:767, 1969.

28. Wynder EL, Schneiderman MA: Exogenous hormones—boon or culprit? J Nat Cancer Inst 51:729, 1973.

29. Casagrande J, Gerkins V, Henderson BE, et al: Brief communication: Exogenous estrogens and breast cancer in women with natural menopause. J Nat Cancer Inst 56:839, 1976.

30. Hoover R, Gray L, Cole P, et al: Menopausal estrogens and breast cancer. N Engl J Med 295:401, 1976.

31. Selikoff IJ, Hammond ED, Churg J: Neoplasm risk associated with occupational exposure to airborne inorganic fibers, in Proceedings of the Tenth International Cancer Congress, Chicago, Year Book Medical, 1970, vol. 5, p. 55.

32. Henderson BE, Gerkins VR, Pike MC: Sexual factors and pregnancy, in Persons at High Risk of Cancer, New York, Academic Press, 1975, p. 270.

33. Mack TM, Henderson BE, Gerkins VR, et al: Reserpine and breast cancer in a retirement community. N Engl J Med 292:1366, 1975.

Panel Discussion:
Risk/Benefit Ratios
of Postmenopausal
Estrogen Administration

Question: The gynecologist can discern what helps his patient avoid menopausal symptoms, but in trying to deal with the problem of osteoporosis, does anyone have any hard data on what appears to be a minimal useful dose of estrogen and a minimal useful duration of estrogen therapy to aid in preventing this complication?

Dr. Morris: The studies in England were performed with ~ 22 μg of mestranol, and that dose is not available in this country for menopausal use. I think the doses available here are too high, so I tell my patients to take a pill twice a week, every other day, or sometimes even once a week. I believe a very small dose is effective in preventing osteoporosis. It won't always stop menopausal symptoms, but I think the dose required to prevent osteoporosis is much smaller.

Dr. Betz: I don't know of a definitive study that shows we can reduce fractures by long-term estrogen treatment.

Dr. Morris: In the studies I quoted, the incidence of fracture was definitely reduced, and I think it is difficult to discount all of the material. Eventually, one will conduct a placebo trial. I believe that there is enough evidence that this kind of approach to the problem should be undertaken with caution. Would you propose that we take a long period of time with women who need estrogens and not put them on hormones?

Dr. Ross: We are currently trying to answer this question retrospectively in our retirement community, but the data are very complex and not yet analyzed completely.

Dr. Silverberg: I recall reading a paper about two years ago that suggested that progesterone therapy might be as effective as estrogen administration in dealing with at least some menopausal symptomatology. Have any other studies indicated that agents other than estrogen might be equally effective in coping with bone mineral loss in osteoporosis?

Dr. Morris: There hasn't been any good study performed with patients on progesterone in this way. Progestagens are tolerated poorly by most patients. Most patients who receive progestagens will bleed, and such therapy can be particularly objectionable due to its long duration (sometimes as long as 6 months) and the fact that it has to be checked by biopsies. When men take progestagens, their basal body temperature rises, they always feel tired, and they lose some of their libido. This study was conducted in Denmark.

No animal species will mate after receiving progestagens, and in monkeys the male may not ejaculate. Thus, I would think progestagens alone would not be well accepted.

Dr. Robboy: One of the implications from the papers presented so far is that the lesions associated with estrogen might not be true endometrial cancer—the lesions have such good prognoses. If one looks at only those patients who have not taken estrogen and matches them grade for grade, stage for stage, what happens to the survival times?

Dr. Silverberg: Dr. Miller showed that in the estrogen-related group, 11 of the 39 patients had real myometrial invasion; six of them were mixed carcinomas, and a few others were what we would consider poorly differentiated (grade II or III) adenocarcinomas. Yet, the recurrence rates were very different, with only one clinical recurrence among the 39 patients who had received estrogen, despite the fact that the follow-up period was the same in both groups. Of course, there has been only a short follow-up period because these cases are mostly recent, but the recurrence rates were very different between the two groups. This finding suggests (although we have to wait until we add the rest of the patients to the study and match them grade for grade and so forth) that even those cases that one might expect to perform poorly in the estrogen-related group do not seem to be doing very poorly, and it raises speculation as to what the cause of that result might be. One wonders whether these tumors need estrogen to "do their thing," and I'm sure that one therapeutic maneuver common to all of these cases is that the patient is taken off estrogen when the diagnosis is made. It is possible that discontinuation of estrogen alone helps the patient as much as the other therapeutic modalities. I think that possibility needs more investigation.

Dr. Robboy: Dr. Morris was pointing out that patients who have well-differentiated tumors and were on estrogen had almost 100% 5-year survival rates.

Dr. Morris: I would be inclined to agree with that; the figures I cited were from Paul Underwood, who said that the patients were an average of 5 years younger and had earlier tumors. But I don't know whether the tumors are, therefore, less bad or whether they detected them earlier. I'm more inclined to favor the latter interpretation.

Dr. Silverberg: In our series, one of our observations was that the duration of symptoms averaged about 4 months in patients who had received estrogen and about 7 months in those who had not received estrogen, so it certainly does seem to be a factor of earlier diagnosis. I am certainly not convinced that earlier diagnosis would change the grade, because I don't see why early diagnosis would be associated with a different histologic grade or histologic type. Certainly, however, it should affect the clinical stage and the likelihood of myometrial invasion and vascular invasion.

Dr. Morris: Both the grade and the stage progress with time. I think it is significant that the patient who received the estrogen prescription must have gone to a doctor unless she borrowed from a girlfriend, and therefore she is in touch with a doctor. The other patients do not want to go to doctors; they try to put it off. If they haven't been told, "if you have some bleeding, come in and see me," they just hope it will go away.

Dr. Silverberg: Does this suggest to you, then, that if the estrogen-related patients had not gone to the doctor, they would have eventually become higher-grade, higher-stage cases? This seems to be a logical conclusion.

Dr. Morris: There is no scientific study to prove it, but I certainly feel that it might be possible.

Dr. Major: Dr. Morris, what is your recommendation for managing a patient on estrogens? Does she need endometrial sampling, endocervical aspirates? For menopausal or postmenopausal patients on estrogen, what do you do before and what do you do after you institute such therapy?

Dr. Morris: In a study from England, endometrial biopsies were obtained before therapy was initiated, and two patients had endometrial carcinoma before they started. However, endometrial biopsy is uncomfortable, and in the patient who is not bleeding, who has no uterine enlargement, and has no symptom that suggests cancer, I would hesitate to obtain such a specimen. I have been told that an endometrial biopsy is like a very severe menstrual cramp or a mild labor pain. The cost of the pathology report is also too great to justify its use except in the presence of the slightest sign of bleeding.

Dr. Major: Then, when you institute estrogen therapy, you don't want the patient to have any withdrawal bleeding.

Dr. Morris: If the patient has withdrawal bleeding, I would discontinue the estrogen and obtain an endometrial biopsy. If the patient telephones and says that she is bleeding, I tell her to stop taking the estrogen and come in and see me in about three weeks, and then I take the endometrial biopsy. This is one reason I hesitate to add progesterone, because it will cause cyclic bleeding for a long period of time.

Dr. Sommers: I would like to quote from the study of Horwitz and Feinstein, reported at the American Society of Epidemiology and the American Society of Clinical Investigation. Who gets the diagnosis of endometrial carcinoma? Somebody who has a D and C. Horwitz and Feinstein collected 6000 D and C cases and found 170 who had carcinoma; all of the others were considered controls. They matched a control to each carcinoma patient by age and by parity. They found a risk ratio for estrogen administration of 1.6. They then divided the cases according to reason for the D and C (bleeders vs. nonbleeders), and the risk ratio was 1.0 for estrogen versus nonestrogen. To me, this figure temporarily cancels out the risk ratio.

Dr. Silverberg: The risk ratio was 1.0 for the bleeders or the nonbleeders?

Dr. Sommers: No, for the use of estrogen versus the nonuse of estrogen, if you divided the cases by bleeders and nonbleeders.

Dr. Silverberg: I don't understand that ratio. It has to be 1.0 for one group or the other. Was it 1.0 for the bleeders and higher for the nonbleeders, or 1.0 for the nonbleeders and higher for the bleeders? If you are changing the risk ratio from 1.6 to 1.0, obviously you are lowering it for one group, and you must be elevating it for the other group. One group must have a risk ratio higher than 1.0.

Dr. Weiss: I can answer that question. These data were presented to us two days ago, and, very strangely, when the data were broken down into smaller groups, both groups had lower risk ratios.

Dr. Silverberg: I'm not a mathematician, but that doesn't make too much sense to me.

Dr. Weiss: I think that the actual comparison is between endometrial cancer patients who showed bleeding compared to the other women with D and Cs without endometrial cancer who also complained of bleeding. The estrogen use in those two groups was identical, thus the risk ratio of 1.0.

  I don't believe that is a very useful study, because it compares two diseases (cancer and bleeding); estrogen is a risk factor for both of them. If, in fact, it causes both diseases, naturally you won't find any difference in estrogen usage. I think we concede that estrogen usage is a cause of postmenopausal bleeding. I'd like to draw another parallel. If you use men with chronic cough as controls for men with lung cancer, you might well find no risk associated with cigarette smoking.

Question: Could someone comment on the management of the patient who is on long-term estrogen and who has a diagnosis at D & C of a very well-differentiated or apparently in situ or focal carcinoma? Do you proceed to hysterectomy, do you discontinue estrogen and repeat the curettage some unspecified or specified amount of time later, or what?

Dr. Major: That is a tough question. At the present time, of course, the accepted treatment for a stage-IA, grade-I lesion is primary hysterectomy alone, without any other adjuvant therapy, and we find that a large number of these patients have no residual cancer. I would think that with this accepted treatment throughout the country today, we would have to institute conservative therapy as a controlled study and obtain a specific informed consent that we are going to delay treatment for this period of time. But it would be very interesting to see what happens. It is conceivable that some of these patients would have no residual cancer and an atrophic endometrium 4–6 weeks later. The others might have a poorly differentiated carcinoma that had been stimulated to exhibit a well-differentiated appearance by the estrogen. Dr. Morris, would you comment on that?

Dr. Morris: I can only treat patients as if they were members of my own family. If my wife had endometrial cancer at curettage and anybody suggested watching her, I would find another physician very quickly. It is true that in a borderline lesion, one can produce regression with progesterone, and I think if you were going to watch the patient very carefully, one could try an interval of progesterone for some special reason. A considerable number of patients eventually have to undergo additional therapeutic intervention for their lesions. With respect to the danger of hysterectomy, it is only in the grossly overweight patient who has just had a coronary or in the patient who is 98 years old that you really worry about it. The average patient has the surgery without complications and is relieved to be rid of an organ that has apparently caused more discomfort than I was aware of, because patients have come in and said, "I feel so much better since the operation." Then I look and find that she had a positive Pap smear and carcinoma in situ at surgery, but she didn't have any complaints. I guess they didn't know what it was like to feel well. I'm sure all of you have had this experience.

Question: What is the current belief regarding the use of parenteral, implantable, and other forms of nonoral estrogen therapy in preventing or alleviating menopausal symptoms, and what role, if any, may these routes of administration have with relation to cancer?

Dr. Betz: My experience with injectables is usually in patients referred to me in whom oral estrogens haven't been adequate. The patient usually has the impression that she doesn't absorb oral estrogens. We have studied many such patients, and invariably they do absorb oral estrogens, so that if they really require injectable estrogens, there are usually other factors involved. Thus, I really don't think injectable estrogen has much utility. Implantable estrogen certainly has been used in a few centers; Dr. Greenblatt has used it for years, and it works very well and lasts months and months, but we lose some of our control over treatment.

Dr. Morris: You use injectables or other techniques when the patient can't swallow; in other words, who wants a needle if she can take a pill? Another problem with injectable Provera is that it remains in the patient for months. I would think that if the patient did develop a problem, you couldn't do anything about it, whereas with pills, you can say, "stop taking them."

Question: Dr. Morris, do you perform mammography before you place a postmenopausal woman on estrogens?

Dr. Morris: I am not a great believer in some of these studies. If the patient doesn't have nodularity in her breasts, I think to give her the x-ray exposure and the $100 charge is unjustified. Mammography is only for the person in whom you wish to follow something that is suspicious.

Dr. Silverberg: Postmenopausal women are already at increased risk of breast cancer by virtue of their age. In all likelihood, you would find a lot of support for the idea that any postmenopausal woman should have a mammogram every so often. How often is open to debate.

Question: Since a certain percentage of women who receive cyclic estrogen will eventually bleed, even on a regimen of 0.3 mg, 21 days on and 7 days off for 2 or

3 years, this bleeding suggests that they probably have accumulated estrogen, because they don't completely deciduate in that one week off back to a non-proliferating state. There are also spurts of endogenous estrogen production. Why do you not concede that these people would have less D & Cs, less chance of developing malignancy, by being deciduated every month with a progestagen? Isn't this therapy safer for a few years than 21 days on and 7 days off?

Dr. Morris: It is perfectly reasonable, but in my experience, there is more bleeding when you begin progestagen administration. Possibly, one should run a certain number of cycles of estrogen alone and then add progestagen periodically. I also think we need a control study to make a comparison with the patient without progesterone. This kind of study would be perfectly acceptable. I don't think there is any convincing evidence that progesterone would cause any side effect, and it might even be beneficial.

Dr. Silverberg: We are essentially talking about a sequential regimen, and some of the data we are going to discuss later might suggest that the sequential regimen does not offer the kind of protection that we might hope it would.

Oral Contraceptives and Endometrial Cancer

Steven G. Silverberg, M.D.

The relationship of oral contraceptive agents to human neoplasms, both benign and malignant, has been the subject of considerable discussion in recent years. Despite numerous investigations on this subject, however, this author believes that we will soon see in this and subsequent discussions that the only conclusive evidence linking these agents to a human neoplasm is related to the benign hepatocellular adenoma.

The results of investigations into other neoplasms, particularly malignant ones, are confusing for several reasons. Perhaps the most important of these reasons is the fact that the oral contraceptive agents only have been used by large numbers of women for less than 15 years. From what we know of generally accepted carcinogenic stimuli, such as ionizing radiation, the period between exposure to the agent and clinical detection of a cancer averages about 10 years. Although these data relate generally to a single rather than continuous exposure, the author believes that they do suggest that all of the data on oral contraceptives certainly will not be available for several more years.

Another obvious reason for the difficulty in appreciating these relationships is the rarity of some of the tumors under investigation. Perhaps the best example is found in the field of endometrial carcinoma, which will be discussed more fully later in this chapter. It is important to remember that, in our recent review of the pertinent literature (1), only 2.4% of patients with endometrial carcinoma were under the age of 40. Since the great majority of oral contraceptive users are in this age range, one would expect to see very few cases of this tumor in oral contraceptive users, and this indeed has been our experience.

The establishment of a control population has been a major problem both in our own studies and in those of other investigators studying different tumors. This problem is complicated by the fact that most medical histories fail to mention whether a patient has taken oral contraceptives, and thus retrospective case review often fails to provide adequate information concerning whether a particular woman should be studied as part of the user or nonuser group. An obvious solution, and one that we have utilized, is to use as controls those women who were seen prior to the period during which oral contraceptives became generally available. This solution, however, poses its own problems as well, because it has been pointed out that the histologic picture of endometrial cancer has changed considerably in the past 30 years (2). In view of this fact, it is a logical conclusion that other clinical and epidemiologic factors in this disease also may have changed, so that oral contraceptive usage is probably not the only variable when one compares patients with endometrial cancer in 1977 with patients with the same disease who were diagnosed in 1957.

Another complicating factor in the analysis of the relationship of oral contraceptives to various tumors is the fact that these agents are indeed heterogeneous, as is the pattern of their usage. Thus, some women use oral contraceptives continuously for a period of 10 or 15 years, while others use them for only a few months, and still others use them intermittently, interspersed with other contraceptive techniques and with pregnancies. Furthermore, the types of estrogen and progestagen, their relative strengths, and their patterns of administration (combined versus sequential) all vary in the different regimens, a fact that has rarely been taken into account in designing and interpreting epidemiologic studies on these agents. Thus, the statement that women taking "the pill" have no greater a risk for the development of a certain type of tumor than do women not using oral contraceptives may actually conceal an increased risk with one type of agent and a decreased risk with another type. This possibility alone leads us to regard almost all earlier studies with a certain degree of suspicion.

With some of these caveats and apologia in mind, let us review what is known of the relation between oral contraceptives and endometrial carcinoma, with emphasis on our studies in this field. Our interest in this problem began in early 1973, when we saw in consultation during a period of a few months three cases of endometrial carcinoma occurring in young women who were taking oral contraceptives. Of particular interest was the fact that two of these women had received only Oracon and that the third had taken both Oracon and several other agents.

When we attempted to review the subject of endometrial cancer in oral contraceptive users in the literature, we drew a complete blank, because no such case had ever been reported. In fact, in several review articles on potential hazards of oral contraceptive administration (3–7), either endometrial carcinoma had not been mentioned at all or it had been suggested that these agents should be protective against the development of this tumor because of their predominantly progestational effect. Thus, we were operating in a vacuum, but we believed that we had made an observation which might turn out to be significant. I presented the histopathologic slides from one of our cases at a workshop at a national meeting of the American Society of Clinical Pathologists and asked the approximately 100 pathologists there if they had ever seen such a case. The response was negative, and so we knew that we were probably dealing with an uncommon problem and probably would not see many more such cases unless we somehow encouraged their referral to us. We also believed that premature publication of our first three cases would be damaging, since it might have created a panic reaction that might not have been justified by subsequent data.

We thus decided that the best thing to do at that time would be to establish a Registry to accumulate more cases. We wanted to study all cases of endometrial cancer occurring in young women taking any type of oral contraceptive, because we could then determine whether the agent (Oracon) that we had seen in association with our first three cases would continue to be overrepresented. We were originally most impressed by the association, because we knew that Oracon was not one of the most popular oral contraceptives. In fact, as we learned later, the sequential agents accounted for only approximately 8% of the oral contraceptive sales in this country, and Oracon for approximately two thirds of that 8%. (The exact figures are somewhat of a trade secret, but I believe that these approximations are reasonable.)

We further decided to limit the Registry to patients who were under 40 years of age at the time of diagnosis. This decision was made essentially for two reasons, one scientific and one practical. The scientific reason was the rarity of endometrial carcinoma in this age group. By studying only cases in these young women, we felt that we could limit somewhat the number of cases that would have occurred spontaneously in which oral contraceptive usage was merely coincidental. The practical reason was that we did not have any special funding for this project, and so we wanted to avoid accessioning so many cases that the load would become unmanageable by Dr. Makowski and myself without any additional resources.

Being somewhat of a babe in the woods in these matters, I telephoned my friend, Dr. Stanley Robboy, who had participated in the establishment of the very successful Diethylstilbestrol Registry in Boston, and enquired as to how one goes about starting a Registry. His response was, "Hang out a shingle that says you are a Registry," and that is exactly what we did. We advertised in medical journals, particularly those in the fields of pathology and obstetrics and gynecology, we made appeals at a couple of national meetings, we sent letters to department chairmen, gynecologic oncologists, and surgical pathologists at all of the medical schools, and we sat back and waited to receive cases.

As one might expect, we received many cases that did not fit our criteria. In some of them, the patient was over 40 years of age. In others, the age was within the acceptable range and the patient did have cancer, but it turned out to be adenocarcinoma or squamous cell carcinoma of the cervix. In yet other cases, the age and the cancer satisfied our criteria, but there was inadequate documentation of oral contraceptive administration. Finally, in yet other cases, our review of the histopathologic slides failed to confirm the diagnosis of endometrial carcinoma, most of these cases being interpreted by us as adenomatous hyperplasia. In the process of accessioning the 30 cases that we reported earlier this year (8), we rejected about 20 cases for one or more of the above reasons.

A few words might be in order at this time about the histologic diagnosis of carcinoma of the endometrium. As a practicing surgical pathologist, with two books and many articles on gynecologic pathology to my credit, I am well aware that many of the recent epidemiologic studies on endometrial cancer have suffered from a lack of quality control in pathology. The use of cases in which histologic material is not reviewed is to be condemned, especially since it is well known that the histologic diagnosis of endometrial carcinoma, particularly the well-differentiated and focal cases, is often controversial. For example, the recent review of Ziel's cases in postmenopausal women by three eminent pathologists revealed a considerable level of disagreement, not only between the panel and the original diagnosis but also among the three members of the panel themselves (9). There is no doubt that our cases might well face the same fate if they were reviewed by several different pathologists. Nevertheless, it should be pointed out that histopathologic confirmation by the author was one of the criteria for the acceptance of a case into the Registry, and several cases were indeed excluded by virtue of their not satisfying the author's criteria for the diagnosis of endometrial carcinoma. Furthermore, our first 21 cases were reviewed by a panel of pathologists convened by the Mead Johnson Company (the manufacturer of Oracon), and only four of these cases were rejected as nonmalignant hyperplasia by these panelists, who were chosen by the company with the greatest hope that they would indeed not be cancer.

Our criteria for the histologic diagnosis of endometrial carcinoma were the same ones that we have defined recently in other sources (10–12). This author believes that the diagnosis is best made architecturally rather than cytologically, because the cells of well-differentiated adenocarcinoma often do not differ significantly from those of adenomatous hyperplasia and are frequently better differentiated and less pleomorphic than are those of atypical hyperplasia. The author demands that evidence of stromal invasion by malignant glands be present, as manifested by one of the following three findings: disappearance of stroma between glands (back-to-back glands), fibrosis of stroma between glands, or necrosis of stroma between glands (Figures 1–3). This evidence of invasion is acceptable, even if it is only focal in an otherwise hyperplastic but benign endometrium. This author does not use the term "adenocarcinoma in situ" to refer to an endometrial lesion, because nobody knows exactly what this term indicates. Thus, the spectrum of its usage in the literature varies from glands

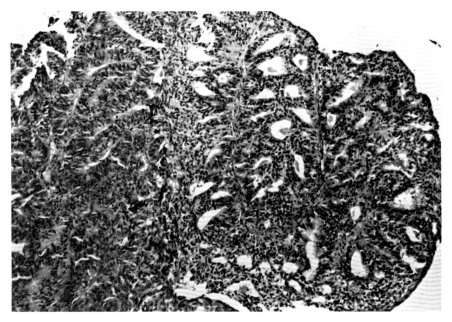

Figure 1. Low-power photomicrograph of curettage specimen from 37-year-old woman who had received Oracon for 8 years. Back-to-back glands without intervening stroma are diagnostic of well-differentiated (grade I) adenocarcinoma.

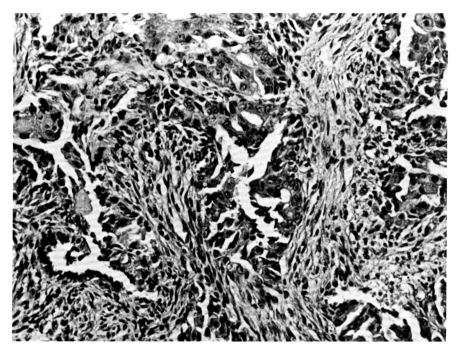

Figure 2. Endometrial adenocarcinoma shows fibrosis of interglandular stroma.

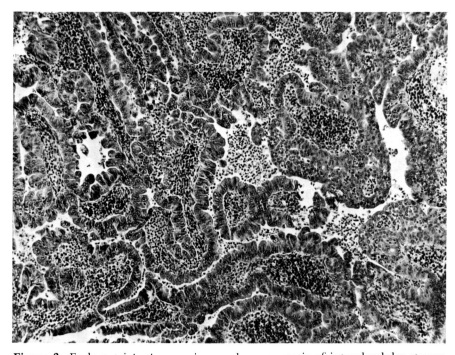

Figure 3. Endometrial adenocarcinoma shows necrosis of interglandular stroma.

that exhibit cellular atypia and cytoplasmic eosinophilia without stromal invasion (13), to small foci of invasive carcinoma as it has been defined above (14), to any carcinoma of the endometrium, no matter how extensive, that does not invade the myometrium (15).

The majority of the tumors in our Registry tended to be both well differentiated and focal. Thus, 22 of the 30 cases were classified as either grade-I adenocarcinoma, adenoacanthoma (adenocarcinoma with squamous metaplasia), or secretory carcinoma. All of these tumors are histologically well differentiated and tend to be associated with a good prognosis. However, it should be pointed out that this picture is not unique to tumors that occur in women who receive oral contraceptives. When we examined a control series of cases of endometrial carcinoma occurring in women under 40 years of age who had not received oral contraceptives, 21 of these 25 cases were similarly placed in the well-differentiated categories mentioned above. The only difference in histology between the Registry cases and the controls was an abundance of cases of pure clear-cell or secretory carcinoma or carcinoma displaying a focal secretory pattern (Figure 4) in the Registry (14 of 29 Registry cases vs. two of 25 controls). Although we tended to attribute this difference to progestational hormonal influence, we noted that four of the 14 Registry patients had discontinued oral contraceptives 8 months to 6 years prior to diagnosis.

As with our cases, when one reviews the literature on endometrial carcinoma in young women, the great majority of cases are recorded as being well differentiated. Fifteen of Bachmann's 25 cases (16) and 10 of Kempson and Pokorny's 15 cases (17) were reported as grade I in a three-grade system. Similarly, 31 of

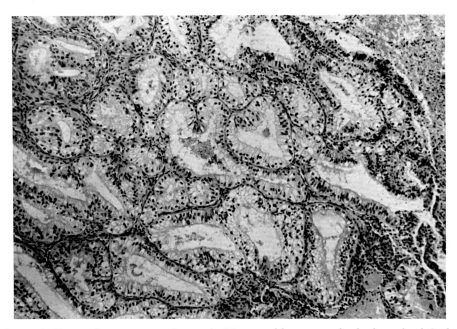

Figure 4. Focus of secretory carcinoma in 35-year-old woman who had received Ortho-Novum for 3 years, followed by Oracon for 5 years. The tumor was elsewhere predominantly an adenoacanthoma.

Dockerty et al.'s 36 cases (18) and 13 of the 16 cases of McGee (19) were reported as grade I or II in a four-grade system, which is generally considered to be equivalent. Thus, although our cases were predominantly well differentiated, this is no reason to be any more suspicious of them than of any other cases seen in women in this age group.

In a similar vein, although about half of our carcinomas were focal lesions in curettage specimens that otherwise usually demonstrated hyperplasia (Figure 5), we do not believe that this factor is an adequate reason to deny their importance. It is certainly true that the majority of these focal lesions can be treated conservatively, and indeed several of them were apparently cured by curettage alone, in that no residual tumor was found in the subsequent hysterectomy specimen or a subsequent D and C. Oral contraception had also been discontinued in these patients after the diagnosis of cancer was made, so it is difficult to determine whether the curettage, the discontinuance of medication, or both was the "curative" agent. Here again, however, it is pertinent to note that in series of endometrial carcinomas in older women, in whom exogenous hormones were probably not a factor (since the cases were diagnosed before the hormone era), approximately 10% of cases had no residual tumor at hysterectomy, even in the absence of prior radiation therapy (20, 21).

The prognosis of these lesions appears to be extremely good. We have only very short follow-up periods on the majority of our cases because of the very recent diagnoses, but, nevertheless, we have seen only one tumor-related death

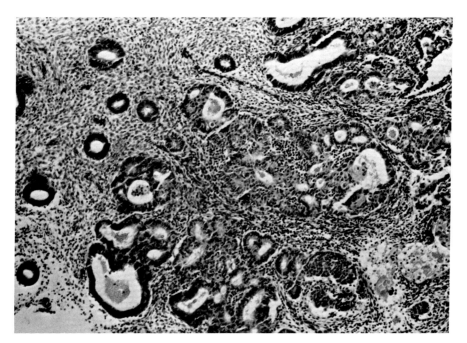

Figure 5. Minute focus of adenocarcinoma in an adenomatous hyperplasia in a 24-year-old woman who had received Oracon for 3 years. Oracon was discontinued, but at age 30, the patient underwent hysterectomy for mixed adenosquamous carcinoma (see Figure 7).

among our 30 patients, in a woman who had received combined agents for a longer period of time than she had received Oracon.

Another indication of tumor aggressiveness is provided by examination of hysterectomy specimens. In the 18 cases in which hysterectomy was performed without prior radiation therapy, only two showed myometrial invasion. Although this figure is low, it does not differ significantly from the incidence of myometrial invasion either in cases in our series without an oral contraceptive history (six of 15) or in cases in the literature in women under 40 years of age (19 of 87). Similarly, the incidence of extrauterine extension or metastasis was extremely low and in many instances probably represented a separate primary lesion rather than true spread. For example, two patients who received Oracon in our Registry had extrauterine lesions that probably represented separate tumors. In one of these women, the lesion was in the endocervix, while in the other it arose in a focus of endometriosis in the vagina (Figure 6). One Registry patient had true metastases in periaortic nodes and the left broad ligament.

In the comparison series that we reviewed from the Armed Forces Institute of Pathology (AFIP), which comprised 25 young patients with endometrial cancer and a negative oral contraceptive history, one case was associated with bilateral ovarian carcinoma of endometrioid type (probably primary, since she is living and well 16 years after treatment by surgery alone), one patient had cervical involvement, and one patient had lymph node metastases. Similarly, in our

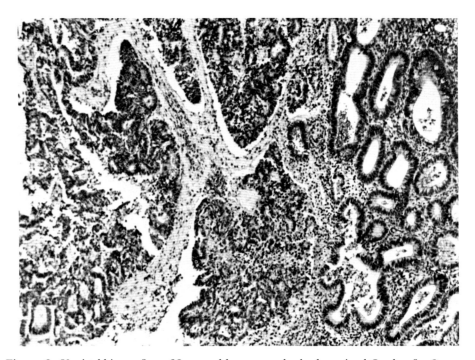

Figure 6. Vaginal biopsy from 32-year-old woman who had received Ovulen for 2 years, followed by Oracon for 7 years. Adenocanthoma of the endometrium was present, with no myometrial invasion evident at hysterectomy. The vaginal lesion is interpreted as a separate primary focus of carcinoma *(left)* arising in endometriosis *(right)*.

literature review, cervical involvement was reported in only two of 87 cases and ovarian tumor in only four.

In the literature series and the AFIP series, in both of which there is better follow-up than in our Registry cases, survival has been excellent. Only eight of 101 patients in the literature have been reported as dead of endometrial cancer, and only two of the 25 AFIP patients died of their tumor. In every case with a lethal outcome that we have been able to review, the tumor was of an unfavorable histologic type (grade-II or -III adenocarcinoma, mixed adenosquamous carcinoma, or clear-cell carcinoma) (22, 23) (Figures 7 & 8), and myometrial invasion, extrauterine spread, or both were seen at the time of hysterectomy. Thus, the risk of death due to cancer in well-differentiated tumors limited to the uterus in this age group appears to be quite minimal, regardless of whether the case is or is not associated with oral contraceptive usage.

This combination of low histologic grade, early clinical stage, lack of local aggressiveness, and excellent prognosis had led some authors to question whether these lesions should indeed be diagnosed as carcinoma. We agree that the biologic malignant potential of these lesions is certainly limited and that treatment should certainly be conservative. Nevertheless, we have persisted in diagnosing them as carcinoma, because we cannot distinguish histologically between these lesions and others that occur in older women and are fully able to invade, metastasize, and kill. This author believes as a pathologist that it is more important to discuss the therapeutic options with the clinician, in view of the patient's age and pattern of hormone usage, than to delude both him and the patient by using a benign name to characterize a lesion that in every other

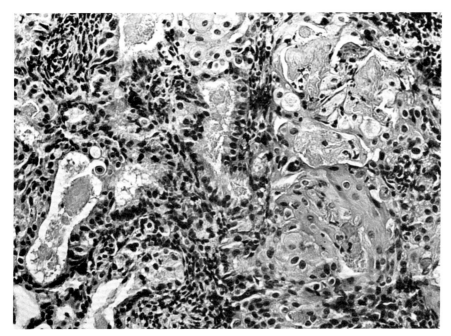

Figure 7. Focus of mixed adenosquamous carcinoma from patient whose history is given in the legend to Figure 5.

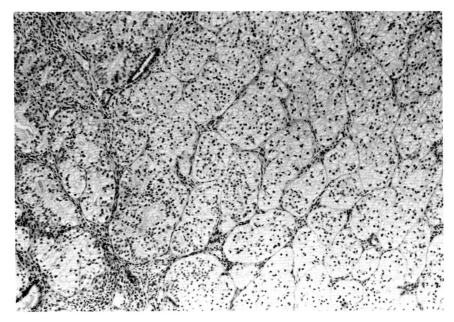

Figure 8. Clear-cell carcinoma in 29-year-old woman who had received Norinyl-2 for 10 months, followed by Oracon for 19 months.

respect satisfies our histologic criteria for carcinoma. The situation is quite analogous to that of papillary carcinoma of the thyroid, in which the tumor is also hormone responsive, the overall survival is also excellent, and the prognosis is also clearly related to the age of the patient. Despite all of these similarities, the author has never heard either a clinician or a pathologist in this field propose that small papillary thyroid cancers in young patients be diagnosed by the pathologist as hyperplasia.

If we are willing, then, to accept the lesions included in our Registry as carcinomas, it will be worthwhile to review their relation to oral contraceptive usage. The bottomline figure is that 20 of the total of 30 patients had taken sequential agents: 19 of these 20 women had received Oracon as their sole or major oral contraceptive, and one had received C-Quens. Nine patients had taken exclusively or predominantly combined agents, and in one the exact nature of the four agents taken was unknown.

This finding of two thirds of the patients receiving sequentials was quite disturbing, in view of the previously mentioned fact that only 8% of oral contraceptive users in this country had received sequentials. However, the data became even more overwhelming when we separated out a group of patients for one or more of the following reasons (Table 1): oral contraceptive therapy instituted at least in part to control abnormal vaginal bleeding rather than strictly for contraception (seven patients), ovarian histology showing polycystic disease consistent with Stein-Leventhal syndrome (six patients), or oral contraceptive history less than 1 year or agents poorly documented (four patients). Of the 11 patients with one or more of these findings, seven had taken combined agents,

Table 1. Principal Oral Contraceptive Agent (OCT) Taken in
Registry Series

	Sequential	*Combined*	*Unknown*
Patients with poor history, OCT for bleeding, or polycystic ovaries	3(1)[a]	7(6)	1(1)
Patients with none of the above	17(2)	2(1)	0

[a] Numbers in parentheses indicate cases in which the OCT was discontinued before the diagnosis of carcinoma.

three had received sequentials, and in one the agents taken were unknown. This distribution is not significantly different from that of oral contraceptive usage in the general population. We believe that in these 11 cases, no serious suspicion of a relationship between oral contraception and carcinoma exists, because of either the short contraceptive history, the fact that in patients with prior bleeding the carcinoma may have been present before the institution of oral contraceptive therapy, and/or the fact that patients with polycystic ovaries are constitutionally predisposed to the development of endometrial cancer (24).

By contrast, of the 19 patients with none of the mitigating circumstances mentioned above, 17 had received predominantly or exclusively sequential agents, and Oracon was the predominant agent in 16 of them. Furthermore, of the nine patients in the entire series who had taken predominantly combined agents, seven had discontinued them prior to the diagnosis of endometrial carcinoma, as opposed to only three of the patients who had taken sequential agents. The duration of oral contraceptive usage in our series ranged from 6 months to 10 years, but, as previously mentioned, women with less than 1 year of usage were assigned to a different subgroup. Thus, sequential users with endometrial carcinoma had a longer oral contraceptive history than did combined agent users with the same diagnosis. The duration of oral contraceptive usage would have no doubt been longer had we accepted patients over 40 years of age into the Registry. Thus, the six patients with endometrial carcinoma reported by Cohen and Deppe (25), four of whom had received Oracon, had reported durations of oral contraceptive use from 5 to 18 years, but five of the six patients were over 40 years of age. Similarly, most of the patients taking Oracon in the combined series of Lyon (26), Kelley et al. (27), and Kaufman et al. (28) were over 40 years of age, and the duration of Oracon usage tended to be longer in these patients.

When Dr. Makowski and the author reported the first 21 patients in our Registry at the meeting of the American College of Obstetricians and Gynecologists in May 1975 [subsequently published in *Cancer* later that year (29)], we were unable to conclude "whether sequential agents somehow predispose their recipients to endometrial cancer, or whether those women who were predestined to develop this tumor are protected against it by combined agents." However, the fact that the changes disappeared in some cases after discontinuance of Oracon suggested the former conclusion, as did the fact that one of our cases occurred in a 36-year-old patient with Turner's syndrome who had been taking Oracon for 10 years. Nevertheless, we strongly believed (and still do) that a controlled study of either cohort or case control type would be necessary in order to be able to choose with certainty between the two alternatives presented above. Thus, we were engaged in planning such a study at the exact time when the announcement was made in February 1976 that the manufacturers of sequential oral contraceptives had decided to withdraw them from the American market. We have subsequently been criticized for having influenced the Food and Drug Administration to pressure the pharmaceutical companies to take this action, but, in fact, our relations with the drug companies were actually far more congenial and mutually informative than were our relations with the FDA. Certainly, we were the first to admit that our conclusions were tentative and required confirmation by further study, and, in fact, this contention was indeed the summary of a presentation that this author made to the FDA in November 1975.

In any event, once the sequentials were off the market, we had nowhere to proceed except to analyze some of the generally accepted risk factors for endometrial carcinoma in our Registry population versus a population of young women with endometrial carcinoma who were nonusers of oral contraceptives. As mentioned above, this analysis was accomplished through the review of cases from the files of the AFIP, with the collaboration of Dr. William D. Roche (8). Our findings are by now well known to all and are recorded in Table 2. We reviewed three risk factors (obesity, gravidity, histologic evidence of polycystic ovarian disease) in four groups of women. First was a literature series, which comprised reported series of women under 40 with endometrial carcinoma, in which the cases dated back far enough to be sure that oral contraceptive usage was minimal. The second group was composed of the 25 cases that we reviewed from the AFIP. The third and fourth groups were our Registry patients who had received combined and sequential agents, respectively. As can be seen in Table 2, the prevalences of obesity, nulligravidity, and polycystic ovarian disease in each of the first three series were remarkably similar and averaged about 50%, thus confirming once again their importance as risk factors in these patients. On the

Table 2. Prevalence of Risk Factors in Endometrial Cancer Patients Under 40 Years of Age Related to Oral Contraceptive Usage

	Obese (%)	Nulligravid (%)	With Polycystic Ovaries (%)
Literature series	54	52	48
AFIP series (no hormones)	60	53	44
Registry series (combined agents)	44	55	44
Registry series (sequential agents)	6	15	14

other hand, only 6% of our sequential users were obese, 15% were nulligravid, and 14% of those in which ovarian pathology was available for review had polycystic ovaries. These differences were all statistically significant and suggested that the sequential users with endometrial carcinoma were certainly not in the constitutionally predisposed group for this disease. Some type of causal relationship thus was suggested, rather than a protective effect of combined oral contraceptives.

This hypothesis fits quite well with what we know about sequential agents in general, Oracon in particular, and recent data concerning the relationship of noncontraceptive estrogenic compounds to endometrial carcinoma. In the combined regimen of oral contraception, estrogen and progestagen are taken together throughout the cycle, and a foreshortened estrogenic or proliferative phase is followed by prolonged secretory and regressive phases in the typical menstrual cycle. In the sequential regimen, on the other hand, estrogen is unopposed by progestagen for the first 14 days of each therapeutic cycle, and histologically a normal or even hyperplastic proliferative phase is followed by shorter periods of secretion and regression (4, 30). Furthermore, the estrogen (ethynylestradiol) used in Oracon has a particularly potent effect on the endometrium (31), while the progestagen (dimethisterone) is particularly weak (32). The partially unopposed stimulation by a particularly strong estrogen thus fits well with what we know of stimulation to the development of endometrial carcinoma by other estrogenic agents, as discussed earlier in this volume.

What, then, are the main conclusions and significant findings of these studies? In addition to the obvious one that scientific investigation should not be conducted in the political arena, there are several other important observations. The first is the confirmation of the fact that different types of estrogen may well have the same end effect or "final common pathway" in terms of their action on the endometrium. The fact that both Premarin and ethynylestradiol are putatively incriminated in the development of endometrial carcinoma suggests that we must be careful in the future in assuming that any one estrogenic product is safer than another. Certainly, these compounds are all metabolized in the body, and we should not be surprised that the end results may be the same.

Second, our study was the first to analyze risks separately for different types of oral contraceptive preparations. As mentioned previously, the "no increased risk" statements about "the pill" made in the past in reference to various disease states may have to be reanalyzed in view of these data. For example, since sequential usage comprised only about 10% of combined agent usage in the past, a relative risk for any disease of 10.0 for sequentials, balanced against one of 0.90 for combined agents, would balance out as 1.0 for "the pill." The same statement could be made for mestranol versus ethynylestradiol, or any of the other different regimens encompassed within the broad spectrum of oral contraceptive usage. This author believes that the lesson learned here is equally applicable to other classes of medications and other therapeutic maneuvers as well.

Finally, we always have to remember the concept of the risk/benefit ratio. Presumably, one of the reasons that the sequential agents were withdrawn from the market so quickly was the fact that many experts did not feel that they really offered a significant therapeutic advantage for contraception over the combined agents. As a nonclinician, the author is not able to evaluate the correctness or incorrectness of this conclusion but believes that the very low incidence of carcinoma in women taking sequentials would have been given less weight had there been more support for a clear-cut therapeutic advantage of these agents.

REFERENCES

1. Silverberg SG: The disease in young women, in *Endometrial Carcinoma and Its Treatment*, Gray LA Sr (ed.), Springfield, Ill., Charles C Thomas, 1977, p. 19.
2. Reagan JW: The changing nature of endometrial cancer. Gynecol Oncol **2:**144, 1974.
3. Craig JM: The pathology of birth control. Arch Pathol **99:**233, 1975.
4. Fechner RE: The surgical pathology of the reproductive system and breast during oral contraceptive therapy. Pathol Annu **6:**299, 1971.
5. Lehfeldt H: Current status of oral contraceptives. Obstet Gynecol Ann **2:**261, 1973.
6. Sperling MA: Complications of systemic oral contraceptive therapy: neoplasm—breast, uterus, cervix and vagina. West J Med **122:**42, 1975.
7. Vessey MP: Thromboembolism, cancer, and oral contraceptives. Clin Obstet Gynecol **17:**65, 1974.
8. Silverberg SG, Makowski EL, Roche WD: Endometrial carcinoma in women under 40 years of age. Comparison of cases in oral contraceptive users and non-users. Cancer **39:**592, 1977.
9. Gordon J, Reagan JW, Finkle WD, et al: Estrogen and endometrial carcinoma: pathological support of original risk estimate. N Engl J Med **297:**570, 1977.
10. Gompel C, Silverberg SG: *Pathology in Gynecology and Obstetrics*. Philadelphia and Toronto, JB Lippincott, 1977, 2nd edit.
11. Silverberg SG: *Surgical Pathology of the Uterus*. New York, John Wiley & Sons, 1977.
12. Silverberg SG: Current concepts in endometrial cancer and hyperplasia. Contemp Ob/Gyn **9:**123, 1977.
13. Buehl IA, Vellios F, Carter JE, et al: Carcinoma *in situ* of the endometrium. Amer J Clin Pathol **42:**594, 1964.
14. Welch WR, Scully RE: Precancerous lesions of the endometrium. Human Pathol **8:**503, 1977.
15. Dallenbach-Hellweg G: *Histopathology of the Endometrium*. New York-Heidelberg-Berlin, Springer-Verlag, 1975, 2nd edit.
16. Bachmann FF: Das Adenokarzinom des Endometriums bei Frauen unter 40 Jahren. Zentr Gynäkol **95:**1729, 1973.
17. Kempson RL, Pokorny GE: Adenocarcinoma of the endometrium in women aged forty and younger. Cancer **21:**650, 1968.
18. Dockerty MB, Lovelady SB, Foust GT: Carcinoma of the corpus uteri in young women. Amer J Obstet Gynecol **61:**966, 1951.
19. McGee WB: Carcinoma of the endometrium in women under 40 years of age. Obstet Gynecol **11:**388, 1958.
20. Nolan JF, Dorough ME, Anson JH: The value of preoperative radiation therapy in stage I carcinoma of the uterine corpus. Amer J Obstet Gynecol **98:**663, 1967.
21. Silverberg SG, DeGiorgi LS: Histopathologic analysis of preoperative radiation therapy in endometrial carcinoma. Amer J Obstet Gynecol **119:**698, 1974.
22. Silverberg SG, Bolin MG, DeGiorgi LS: Adenoacanthoma and mixed adenosquamous carcinoma of the endometrium: a clinicopathologic study. Cancer **30:**1307, 1972.
23. Silverberg SG, DeGiorgi LS: Clear cell carcinoma of the endometrium: clinical, pathologic, and ultrastructural findings. Cancer **31:**1127, 1973.
24. Fechner RE, Kaufman RH: Endometrial adenocarcinoma in Stein-Leventhal syndrome. Cancer **34:**444, 1974.

25. Cohen CJ, Deppe G: Endometrial carcinoma and oral contraceptives. Obstet Gynecol **49:**390, 1977.

26. Lyon FA: The development of adenocarcinoma of the endometrium in young women receiving long-term sequential oral contraception: report of 4 cases. Amer J Obstet Gynecol **123:**299, 1975.

27. Kelley HW, Miles PA, Buster JE, et al: Adenocarcinoma of the endometrium in women taking sequential oral contraceptives. Obstet Gynecol **47:**200, 1976.

28. Kaufman RH, Reeves KO, Dougherty CM: Severe atypical endometrial changes and sequential contraceptive use. J Amer Med Ass **236:**923, 1976.

29. Silverberg SG, Makowski EL: Endometrial carcinoma in young women taking oral contraceptive agents. Obstet Gynecol **46:**503, 1975.

30. Kistner RW: Endometrial alterations associated with estrogen and estrogen-progestin combinations, in *The Uterus,* Norris HJ (ed.), Baltimore, Williams & Wilkins, 1973, p. 227.

31. Delforge JP, Ferin J: A histometric study of two estrogens: ethinyl-estradiol and its 3-methyl-ether derivative (mestranol); their comparative effect upon the growth of the human endometrium. Contraception **1:**57, 1970.

32. Dickey RP, Stone SC: Progestational potency of oral contraceptives. Obstet Gynecol **47:**106, 1976.

Effect of Oral Contraceptive Use on the Risk of Human Breast and Cervical Cancer

Bruce V. Stadel, M.D., M.P.H.

Oral contraceptives were first marketed in the United States in June 1960, when Enovid (10 mg of norethynodrel and 150 μg of mestranol) was introduced. By 1965, 15.3% of currently married American women between the ages of 15 and 44 reported current oral contraceptive use when interviewed. This figure grew to 25.1% by 1973, over 6.5 million women (1).

At first glance, such widespread exposure to oral contraceptives, coupled with the relatively high incidence of breast and cervical cancer and its precursors among women in the United States, would seem to make assessment of the effects of oral contraceptive use on the risk of these cancers comparatively simple. This is true to a limited extent, but important questions concerning extended oral contraceptive use, latency of the effects of use, and interactions between oral contraceptive effects and the effects of other known or hypothesized risk factors for these cancers remain unresolved. In the study of cervical cancer, lack of agreement concerning the classification of precursors to invasive carcinoma and uncertainty concerning the rate of irreversible progression from precursor lesions to invasive carcinoma have also posed problems in the interpretation of published data.

BREAST CANCER

The published literature concerning the basic epidemiology of breast cancer is vast; fortunately, most information published prior to the present decade was reviewed thoroughly by MacMahon et al. in 1973 (2). Published studies concerning the effects of oral contraceptive use on the risk of breast cancer are by

89

contrast comparatively few. Nevertheless, important questions concerning the possibility of increased breast cancer risk among certain subgroups of oral contraceptive users have been raised. To place these questions in perspective, it may be useful to review briefly some central features of the basic epidemiology of breast cancer.

Basic Epidemiology of Breast Cancer (2)

The major known risk factors for human breast cancer are geographic area of residence, age, age at menarche, age at first birth, age at natural menopause, oophorectomy and age at oophorectomy, history of benign breast neoplasia, and family history of breast cancer.

The international variations in breast cancer incidence are quite large: rates are five to six times higher in North America and Northern Europe than in most areas of Asia and Africa. Southern Europe and South America have intermediate rates. Areas with lower rates also appear to have a lower proportion of the more aggressive histologic types of breast cancer and better survival for women with specific histologic types.

These international variations in breast cancer incidence appear to be due to environmental factors rather than to differences in genetics or reproductive behavior. Differences in fat (3) and iodine (4) intake have been hypothesized as explanations for these variations, but these hypotheses have not been tested.

Most of the known risk factors for human breast cancer appear to be mediated through some aspect of estrogen production or metabolism. Thus, breast cancer risk has been reported to increase with decreasing age at menarche and with increasing age at natural menopause. Similarly, oophorectomy has been reported to lower risk; the effect is greater when oophorectomy occurs at a comparatively early age.

The international differences in breast cancer risk mentioned above may also be mediated through differences in estrogen production and metabolism. Higher-risk North American women excrete more estrogen in the urine than do their lower-risk Asian counterparts, with a lower estriol to estrone plus estradiol ratio (5). Also, women of Asian descent living in an area influenced heavily by North American culture (Hawaii) exhibit breast cancer rates and urinary estrogen excretion patterns intermediate between those of Asian and North American women (6).

Age at first full-term birth is a powerful predictor of breast cancer risk; a full-term birth prior to age 18 is associated with only about one third of the breast cancer risk associated with a first full-term birth at age 35 or older. This apparent protective effect of a comparatively early first full-term birth may be limited to certain histologic types of breast cancer. The mechanism may involve alterations in estrogen metabolism (7).

Breast cancer risk is apparently increased among women with a family history of breast cancer, but it is uncertain whether this increased risk is due to genetic or familial phenomena.

Fibrocystic disease of the breast ("cystic mastitis, chronic cystic mastitis") has been reported to be a risk factor for breast cancer (8). This issue is complex, because fibrocystic disease may, in fact, be a spectrum of entities with differing biologic meanings. For example, Black et al. have reported that some women with this form of breast disease exhibit ductal atypia and that breast cancer risk is related to the degree of ductal atypia present (9).

This brief survey of the basic epidemiology of breast cancer illustrates the complex web of factors that appear to be involved in the etiology of breast cancer and that bear on efforts to estimate meaningfully the effect of oral contraceptive use on the risk of this disease.

Effect of Oral Contraceptive Use on Breast Cancer Risk
(Tables 1 & 2)

During the past eight years, reports from four case control (10–13) and three cohort studies (14–16) concerning the effect of oral contraceptive (OC) use on breast cancer risk have appeared in the English language literature.

Three of the case control studies reported no evidence of an effect of OC use on breast cancer risk (10–12), while one (13) reported evidence of increased risk among 1) women with a first birth at over 25 years of age and a history of OC use prior to first birth (relative risk = 13.4; p = 0.02), 2) women with a history of a biopsy diagnosis of benign breast disease prior to the development of breast cancer *and* a history of more than 6 years of OC use (relative risk = 11.8; p = 0.04), and 3) current OC users (relative risk = 1.5; p = 0.04) and 4) women with a history of from 2 to 4 years of total OC use (relative risk = 1.8; p = 0.03).

On examination, it is evident that only two of these four case control studies involved substantial numbers of women sufficiently young to have used OCs extensively (12, 13) (Table 1). Only one of these two studies evaluated the use of OCs prior to first birth and among women with a prior biopsy diagnosis of benign breast disease as separate issues; thus, these findings currently stand alone (13). The other of these two studies did evaluate breast cancer risk among current OC users; no effect was reported (12).

The three cohort studies from which data concerning the effect of OC use on breast cancer risk have been published thus far involve too few cases of breast cancer for stable risk estimates and far too few for evaluation of interactions between OC use and other known breast cancer risk factors (14–16) (Table 2).

Benign Breast Neoplasia, Breast Cancer, and Oral Contraceptive Use

An apparent paradox exists in the published data concerning the effect of OC use on the risk of benign breast neoplasia, the relationship of benign breast neoplasia to breast cancer, and the effect of OC use on the risk of breast cancer.

Fibrocystic disease of the breast has been repeatedly reported to be a risk factor for breast cancer, and OC use is believed to reduce the risk of fibrocystic disease of the breast (17). However, Paffenbarger et al. (13) estimated a relative risk for breast cancer of 11.8 for more than 6 years of OC use among women with a biopsy diagnosis of benign breast disease prior to the development of breast cancer.

Paffenbarger et al. (13) do not state what proportion of the OC use among these women with a biopsy diagnosis of benign breast disease prior to the

Table 1. Case Control Studies of Breast Cancer That Refer to Oral Contraceptive Exposure

Investigator and Year	Nature of Study	Matching Factors	Exclusions	Age (years)	Number of Cases	OC Use Among Controls (%)			Further Information Available Concerning Duration of Use	Evidence of an Effect of OC Use on Breast Cancer Risk
						Never Used	<2 yrs	>2 yrs		
Arthes et al. (10) 1971	Hospital based	Age (within 5 years) Race Ever vs. never married Hospital pay status	Prior diagnosis of a breast lesion	15–75	119 (46 <50 years old)	68 (Includes OC, Menopausal Estrogen, or Any Other Female Hormone Use Within 10 Years Prior to Study)	18	13	< 2 Years divided as 0–1 and 1–2	None for ever use, 0–1 years use, 1–2 years use, 2+ years use (any female hormone within 10 years prior to study)
BCDSP (11) 1973	Hospital based	City (Boston) Age (5-year intervals) Year (1972)	Prior diagnosis of a breast lesion Contraindications to OC use	20–44	23	80	20		None	Only three cases had ever used OCs

Study	Type	Matching variables	Exclusions	Age					Duration categories	Results
Vessey et al. (12) 1975	Hospital based	Hospital and interval of admission Age (5-year intervals) Currently married Parity (0, 1, 2–3, 3+)	Never married	16–45	322	62	24	14	< 2 Years divided (by months) as 0–3, 4–12, 12–24, 25+	None for current use, interval since first use, or for 0–3 months of use, 4–12 months use, 12–24 months use, 25+ months use
Paffenbarger et al. (13) 1977	Hospital based	Hospital and interval of admission Age (5-year intervals) Race (black vs. white) Religion (Catholic vs. non-Catholic)	Race other than black or white Nonresident of area Contraindications to OC use	15–49	452	54	22	22	2–4 years = 6% 4–8 years = 13% 8+ years = 3%	Increased risk among women with: Use prior to first birth Extended use and benign breast disease prior to development of cancer Current use, 2–4 years use (see text)

93

Table 2. Cohort Studies of OC Users: Breast Cancer

Investigator and Year	Nature of Study	Age (years)	Number of Women at Enrollment		Exclusions	Women-years of Observation				Standardized Risk by Years of OC Use (number of cases)			
			Ever Users	Never Users		Users	Ex Users	Never Users	Total	0	0-1	1-2	2+
RCGP (14) 1974 (subjects enrolled from 1968 to 1969)	Practice-based cohort	15–49	23,611	22,766	Unmarried or not living as married	34,875	9803	42,306	86,984	1.0 (16)	1.1 (11 current users; 4 ex-users)		
Ory et al. (15) 1976 (subjects enrolled in 1970)[a]	Population-based cohort	25–49	18,646	50,491	Prior diagnosis of breast disease	40,368	NA[b]	109,310	146,678	1.0 (115)	0.6 (12)		0.7 (10)
Vessey et al. (16) 1976 (subjects enrolled from 1968 to 1974)[a]	Clinic-based cohort	25–39	9653	IUD 3162 Dia-phragm 4217	Unmarried, nonwhite, British; History of breast disease	31,076	NA	IUD 10,014 Dia-phragm 14,739	55,829	1.0 IUD (4) Dia-phragm (5)	0.38[c]–0.53[d] (5)		

[a] Changes in contraceptive status between entry into cohort and disease event *not* considered in the analysis. Adherence to method at entry appears large enough that bias thus introduced would be small.

[b] Issue not addressed.

[c] OC vs. IUD.

[d] OC vs. diaphragm.

development of breast cancer occurred before the biopsy diagnosis. It is possible that OC use might suppress fibrocystic disease with low grades of ductal atypia to a greater extent than disease with high grades of atypia. If so, women undergoing a breast biopsy after extensive OC use would be a selected subgroup at higher risk for breast cancer than would women undergoing a breast biopsy in the absence of extensive prior OC use. It is also possible that extensive OC use after the development of fibrocystic disease might tend to accelerate the development of cancer. In this regard, it seems appropriate to note that breast cancer risk among women receiving menopausal estrogen therapy has been reported to be increased, but only after very extended use (18). These possibilities are speculative and will remain so until sufficient data are collected to clarify this situation.

CERVICAL CANCER AND ITS PRECURSORS

Dysplasia, carcinoma in situ, and invasive carcinoma of the cervix have been the subject of myriad epidemiologic, clinical, and experimental investigations. However, reference to a comparatively small number of studies is sufficient to illustrate the problems that encumber efforts to estimate the effects of OC use on the risks of these entities.

Basic Epidemiology of Cervical Cancer and Its Precursors

Overwhelming epidemiologic evidence supports the concept that carcinoma in situ and invasive carcinoma of the cervix are venereal diseases. Specifically, risks of these forms of neoplasia have been inversely correlated to age at first coitus and directly to number of sexual partners (19). Coital transmission of a carcinogen is apparent, and herpes hominis type-II virus has been considered a plausible agent by many investigators, although this hypothesis remains controversial (20, 21).

Although venereal transmission of a carcinogen appears to be the central event in the development of carcinoma in situ and invasive carcinoma of the cervix, endocrine factors may play an accessory role. This is suggested by the observation that the incidence of cervical cancer and the prevalence of atypical cervical hyperplasia and preinvasive cancer increase with age until menopause, and then decline. Also, women with squamous dysplasia, carcinoma in situ, and invasive carcinoma of the cervix show more evidence of endogenous estrogen activity, as judged from the appearance of vaginal epithelial cells, than do normal controls (22).

The etiology of cervical cancer is commonly believed to involve a progression from dysplasia through carcinoma in situ to invasive carcinoma. Three observations tend to temper this theory.

First, a marked similarity between the epidemiologic characteristics of women with carcinoma in situ and invasive carcinoma of the cervix suggests a common etiology. Only a portion of women with cervical dysplasia appear to share these characteristics, however, suggesting that some cervical dysplasia may not be etiologically related to carcinoma in situ and invasive carcinoma. For example, Thomas (22) has reported that marital instability and first childbirth out of wedlock are associated more strongly with carcinoma in situ of the cervix than with cervical dysplasia. Factors of this type have previously been reported to be associated with invasive cervical carcinoma and are believed to reflect the pattern of sexual activity previously mentioned.

Second, while carcinoma in situ appears to be a precursor to invasive cervical carcinoma, the net rate of irreversible progression does not appear to be well established. Published estimates range from 10 to 100% (23). This wide variation may reflect differences in diagnostic criteria for cervical carcinoma in situ.

Third, there appears to be considerable variation among pathologists concerning the diagnosis of carcinoma in situ of the cervix. In one study, a 10-fold difference in the rate of this diagnosis occurred when two pathologists familiar with cervical pathology independently read the same set of 85 slides (24).

Effect of Oral Contraceptive Use on the Risk of Cervical Cancer and Its Precursors

More than 30 epidemiologic studies of the effect of OC use on the risk of cervical cancer and its precursors have been tabulated (25). These studies include one clinical trial in which women were assigned randomly to either OCs or conventional means of contraception (26), three large studies of the prevalence of abnormal cervical cytology among OC users and nonusers (27–29), four case control studies of women with dysplasia, carcinoma in situ, and invasive carcinoma of the cervix (24, 30–32), and three cohort studies of OC users and nonusers (16, 33, 34), which will suffice to provide considerable perspective on the current state of knowledge concerning the effect of OC use on the risk of cervical cancer and its precursors.

A Randomized Clinical Trial of Oral Contraceptives
In 1973, Fuertes de la Haba et al. (26) reported the results of a randomized clinical trial in which 4846 women were assigned to OCs and 4788 were assigned to conventional means of contraception. Changing cytologic status was compared for the two groups. A total of 2249 women changed status at least once, 1225 at least twice, and 690 changed status three times. The authors concluded that there was no significant difference in the patterns of progression and regression of cervical cytologic status when OC users and users of conventional means of contraception were compared. However, Ory et al. (24) have noted that the authors arrived at this conclusion by grouping all women whose cytologic status changed from one diagnostic category to another, regardless of whether they went from normal to atypical or from dysplasia to carcinoma in situ. Ory et al. (24) further observed that the progression rate of women with Papanicolaou smears of class III or higher was twice as large for OC users as for nonusers.

Prevalence of Abnormal Cervical Cytology
Among Oral Contraceptive Users and Nonusers
Three studies of the prevalence of cervical abnormal cervical cytology have revealed no consistent evidence that abnormal cervical cytology is more preva-

lent among OC users than among nonusers (27–29). Berget and Weber (27) reviewed data derived from the 1967–9 screening of 13,125 women between 30 and 50 years of age in Maribo District, Denmark (85% of the eligible female population). Eleven percent of the women screened had used OCs; the average duration of use was 24 months. They observed no overall differences in the prevalence of cervical dysplasia, carcinoma in situ, or invasive carcinoma for OC users as compared to users of other contraceptive methods. Adjustment for age (5-year intervals), parity, age at first pregnancy, and socioeconomic status again revealed no overall difference between OC users and users of other contraceptive methods, but a significantly higher prevalence of abnormal cervical cytology among middle class OC users than among nonusers was noted.

Kirkland and Stanley (28) reviewed the records of 49,798 women screened by a cytology service in Australia. A total of 26,286 OC users were compared with 23,512 nonusers of similar age and parity; 306 cases of carcinoma in situ and 87 cases of invasive carcinoma of the cervix were identified among the 49,798 women. The prevalence of carcinoma in situ of the cervix among OC users under 30 years of age who had two or more children was 2.3 times greater than that among similar nonusers. However, the prevalence of carcinoma in situ was two times greater among nonusers over 40 years of age who had two or more children than that among similar users. Also, the prevalence of invasive cervical carcinoma among women over 30 years of age was 2.9 times greater among nonusers than among women users.

Finally, Miller (29) compared 2394 OC users with an equal number of age- (within 2 years) and race-matched nonusers. The average duration of OC use among the users was 49.1 months. No difference in the prevalence of abnormal cervical cytology was found for any age group.

Case Control Studies of Dysplasia, Carcinoma in Situ, and Invasive Carcinoma of the Cervix

In 1972, Worth and Boyes (30) reported the results of a case control study of 310 women in British Columbia aged 20–29 who had preinvasive cervical cancer. Of these 310 women, 308 were diagnosed as carcinoma in situ. Oral contraceptive use among these women was compared to that among 682 age-matched controls (5-year intervals). Nulliparity was less common and mean parity higher for cases than for controls, but the mean ages at first pregnancy for cases and controls who had been pregnant did not differ appreciably. More cases than controls had been married, and more had been separated or divorced. Mean ages at first marriage for cases and controls who had been married were similar.

Cases and controls were similar with respect to age at first contraceptive use, mean interval between first contraceptive use and entry into the study, "ever use" of OCs, and mean duration of OC use.

Thomas (31) also reported a case control study in 1972. A total of 378 white women aged 15–50 with cervical cytology status of Papanicolaou class III, IV, or V were compared with 360 controls selected on the basis of a one in 30 probability sample of white women aged 15–50, living in the same Maryland county as the cases, who had Pap smears during the interval in which the cases were ascertained (1965–9). Cases of dysplasia and carcinoma in situ were compared to controls concerning 14 epidemiologic variables (including OC use). After extensive analysis, Thomas concluded that the study revealed no evidence that women who used either sequential or combination OCs for a mean duration of 20 months developed cervical dysplasia or carcinoma in situ within 2–3 years after initial use at a rate different from that of women who did not use OCs. It is interesting to note that the risk of cervical carcinoma in situ for OC users relative to that for nonusers was 0.58 (after adjustment for 13 other variables). This finding, while not statistically significant, suggests a negative association between OC use and the risk of development of cervical carcinoma in situ.

Two case control studies of cervical cancer and its precursors appeared in the 1977 literature. Boyce et al. (32) compared 689 women with carcinoma in situ or invasive carcinoma of the cervix with 689 controls matched for age, ethnic origin, socioeconomic status, age at first coitus, and age at first pregnancy. Cases and controls were found to be similar with regard to "ever use" of OCs, type of OC used (containing mestranol vs. containing ethynylestradiol) and mean duration of OC use. Although the study was highly matched in design, a matched-pairs analysis was not used in this presentation of the data. Further analysis by matched pairs is being planned.

Ory et al. (24) conducted a case control study within a population of women who attended an inner-city family planning clinic in Atlanta, Georgia during the period 1967–72. The study was confined to black women between the ages of 15 and 44 whose records revealed either OC or intrauterine device (IUD) use; users of other methods of contraception were excluded. Furthermore, only women with at least three Pap smears on file were included.

The cases comprised 854 black women who developed cervical dysplasia and 147 who developed cervical carcinoma in situ during the years 1970–2, following at least two normal and no abnormal Pap smears. Cases were included only if the initial smear diagnosis was confirmed by biopsy within 1 year. Controls comprised 8553 black women with a normal Pap smear during the years 1970–2 and at least two prior normal and no abnormal Pap smears.

To control confounding, 10 variables were summarized into a multivariate risk score. These variables included age, educational status, marital status, age at first birth, parity, contraceptive method at the time of case and control ascertainment, frequency of prior Pap smears, and other factors that might be related to both contraceptive choice and disease risk. Using this multivariate score, three strata of risk for dysplasia and carcinoma in situ of the cervix were created. Standardized relative risks for OC use were computed over the three strata. The risk of cervical carcinoma in situ for OC users as compared to nonusers was estimated to be 1.3 for 1–12 months of use, 2.5 for 13–24 months of use, 2.6 for 24–36 months of use, and 4.7 for more than 36 months of use. A statistical test for increasing risk with increasing duration of OC use was highly significant.

To test the biologic meaning of these findings, Ory et al. (24) submitted 85 tissue sections bearing a hospital diagnosis of carcinoma in situ to two pathologists generally accepted as experts in cervical pathology. One agreed with 85% of the hospital diagnoses, but the other agreed with only 14%. The latter read 54% of these tissue sections as moderate dysplasia.

Cohort Studies of Oral Contraceptive Users
In 1973, Malamed and Flehinger (33) reported the incidence of "all precancerous lesions" and carcinoma in situ among OC users, IUD users, and diaphragm

users. Each of 911 IUD users and 1015 diaphragm users was matched to three OC users for age group, ethnic group, age at first pregnancy, number of live births, and family income. All study subjects had had at least two normal Pap smears prior to enrollment.

These cohorts of contraceptive users were observed for 38 months, with steady attrition of subjects from all categories. No statistically significant difference in the incidence of either cervical carcinoma in situ or "all precancerous lesions" was apparent for either the OC versus diaphragm cohort or for the OC versus IUD cohort. It is interesting to note, however, that the incidence of carcinoma in situ was about twofold higher for OC users than for either diaphragm or IUD users. This result was not statistically significant, but the size of the study was insufficient to distinguish small differences in incidence rates (diaphragm vs. OC, 1.4 vs. 2.8 per 1000 women-years; IUD vs. OC, 0.6 vs. 1.4 per 1000 women-years).

In 1976, Vessey et al. (16) reported rates of dysplasia and carcinoma in situ of the cervix in interim results from observation of a cohort of 17,032 British women who were 25–39 years of age when enrolled during the interval 1968–74. Among these women, 56.6% used OCs on entry, 24.8% used diaphragms, and 18.6% used IUDs. The interim analysis was based on women-years of observation according to method of contraception in use on entry into the study; crossover had thus far been small. Loss to follow-up had also been small. The incidence of cervical dysplasia for OC and IUD users was similar: 0.31 per 1000 women-years for OC users and 0.21 per 1000 women-years for IUD users. The incidence of cervical carcinoma in situ followed the same pattern: 0.45 per 1000 women-years for OC users and 0.43 per 1000 women-years for IUD users. No case of either condition had been observed in diaphragm users; the difference between diaphragm users and OC or IUD users was highly significant statistically, suggesting that diaphragm use protects against cervical dysplasia and carcinoma in situ.

In 1977, Stern et al. (34) published the results of over 7 years of observation of a cohort of oral contraceptive users and nonusers. The study subjects were selected from approximately 11,000 women who enrolled in Los Angeles Family Planning Clinics during the years 1967–71. Only women with no prior history of oral contraceptive use or of an illness that might bias contraceptive choice were considered eligible. Three hundred women with cervical dysplasia were identified from among the approximately 6000 women who satisfied these criteria. Another 300 women with normal Pap smears were identified concurrently and followed in the same manner as the women with cervical dysplasia.

The study subjects were examined by Pap smear at 2 months, 6 months, and then every 6 months. All Pap smear evaluations were performed without knowledge of the subjects' contraceptive status. Rates of progression of cervical dysplasia to carcinoma in situ were compared for OC users and nonusers. More than 90% of the OC nonusers used IUDs. The data were analyzed by life table procedures; women who changed contraceptive method or became pregnant were excluded from the time these events occurred. Dropout rates and reasons for dropout or exclusion did not appear to differ according to the contraceptive method used.

The data from this study suggest that:

1. Progression from cervical dysplasia to carcinoma in situ among young

women (average age 23 years) is, in general, slow. During over 800 women-years of observation of women with cervical dysplasia at initiation of the study, only 13 cases of carcinoma in situ appeared. The majority of these women were using OCs during this observation period; if OC use increases the rate of progression from cervical dysplasia to carcinoma in situ, this is an overestimate of the natural rate of progression.

2. Oral contraceptive use does not appear to increase the incidence of abnormal cervical cytology among women with normal Pap smears at the time they begin oral contraceptive use. This conclusion is based on observation of a cohort too small to provide evidence of small changes in incidence rates.

3. Extended OC use (> 6 years) appears to increase the rate of conversion of cervical dysplasia to carcinoma in situ among women with dysplasia at the time they begin OC use by several-fold. This conclusion is based on observation of a cohort of women that underwent steady attrition during over 7 years of observation; the validity of the conclusion rests on the assumption that this attrition process introduced no bias.

DISCUSSION AND CONCLUSIONS

Although oral contraceptives were introduced in the United States in 1960, usage did not become widespread for several years (1). It has therefore only recently become possible to evaluate the effect of OC usage on the risk of breast and cervical cancer in a comprehensive manner.

Breast Cancer

Data concerning the effect of OC use on breast cancer risk have been reported from four case control studies (10–13) and three cohort studies (14–16). No overall increase in breast cancer risk for OC users has been observed. Only one study (13), however, has specifically analyzed possible interactions between OC use and previously reported breast cancer risk factors, such as age at first birth and benign breast disease. This study suggests that OC use may increase breast cancer risk among certain subgroups of women and indicates the need for further study.

Cervical Cancer and Its Precursors

The available data regarding the effect of OC use on the risk of cervical cancer and its precursors are confusing and inconclusive. Most of these data do not control directly for possible confounding between OC use and age at first coitus and number of sexual partners. Use of such variables as socioeconomic status, marital status, and parity in an effort to control indirectly for possible confounding between OC use and sexual behavior may be insufficient.

Few studies have evaluated the effect of OC use on the risk of cervical cancer and its precursors separately for women with previously reported cervical cancer risk factors. Such an evaluation seems desirable, because OC use might affect risk only among women exposed to a venereally transmitted carcinogen prior to OC use.

Finally, virtually all available studies of the effect of OC usage on the risk of cervical cancer and its precursors have had cervical dysplasia or carcinoma in situ as their biologic endpoint. Diagnostic criteria for these lesions appear to vary widely, as do estimates of their invasive potential. These issues must be resolved if future studies are to provide meaningful information regarding the effect of OC use on the risk of invasive cervical cancer.

The information currently available is insufficient to warrant the conclusion that OC use affects the risk of either breast or cervical cancer. These data are sufficient, however, to indicate a need for further studies of these issues.

REFERENCES

1. Westhoff CF: Trends in contraceptive practice: 1965–1973. Family Planning Perspect **8**:54, 1976.

2. MacMahon B, Cole P, Brown J: Etiology of human breast cancer: a review. J Nat Cancer Inst **50**:21, 1973.

3. Carroll KK, Gammel EB, Plunkett ER: Dietary fat and mammary cancer. Can Med Ass J **98**:540, 1968.

4. Stadel BV: Dietary iodine and risk of breast, endometrial, and ovarian cancer. Lancet **1**:890, 1976.

5. MacMahon B, Cole P, Brown JB, et al: Urine estrogen profiles of Asian and North American women. Int J Cancer **14**:161, 1974.

6. Dickenson LE, MacMahon B, Cole P, et al: Estrogen profiles of Oriental and Caucasian women in Hawaii. N Engl J Med **291**:1211, 1974.

7. Cole P, Brown JB, MacMahon B: Estrogen profiles of parous and nulliparous women. Lancet **2**:596, 1976.

8. Monson RR, Yen S, MacMahon B: Chronic mastitis and carcinoma of the breast. Lancet **2**:224, 1976.

9. Black MM, Barclay TH, Cutler SJ, et al: Association of atypical characteristics of benign breast lesions with subsequent risk of breast cancer. Cancer **29**:338, 1972.

10. Arthes FG, Sartwell PE, Lewison EF: The pill, estrogens, and the breast. Cancer **28**:1391, 1971.

11. Boston Collaborative Drug Surveillance Program: Oral contraceptives and venous thromboembolic disease, surgically confirmed gall-bladder disease, and breast tumours. Lancet **1**:1400, 1973.

12. Vessey MP, Doll R, Jones K: Oral contraceptives and breast cancer. Lancet **1**:941, 1975.

13. Paffenbarger RS Jr, Fasal E, Simmons ME, et al: Cancer risk as related to use of oral contraceptives during fertile years. Cancer **39**:1887, 1977.

14. Royal College of General Practitioners: *Oral Contraceptives and Health.* New York, Pitman, 1974.

15. Ory H, Cole P, MacMahon B, et al: Oral contraceptives and reduced risk of benign breast diseases. N Engl J Med **294**:419, 1976.

16. Vessey M, Doll R, Peto R, et al: A long-term follow-up study of women using different methods of contraception—an interim report. J Biosoc Sci **8**:373, 1976.

17. Cole PT: Oral contraceptives and breast neoplasia. Cancer **39**:1906, 1977.

18. Hoover R, Gray LF Sr, Cole P, et al: Menopausal estrogens and breast cancer. N Engl J Med **295**:401, 1976.

19. Rotkin ID: Adolescent coitus and cervical cancer: associations of related events with increased risk. Cancer **27**:603, 1967.

20. Adam E, Rauls EW, Melnick JL: The association of herpes virus type 2 infection and cervical cancer. Preventive Med **3**:122, 1974.

21. Nahmias AJ, Naib ZM, Josey WE: Epidemiologic studies relating genital herpetic infection to cervical carcinoma. Cancer Res **34**:1111, 1974.

22. Thomas DB: An epidemiologic study of carcinoma in situ and squamous dysplasia of the uterine cervix. Amer J Epidemiol **98**:10, 1973.

23. Green GH, Donovan JW: The natural history of cervical carcinoma in situ. J Obstet Gynaecol Brit Comm **77**:1, 1970.

24. Ory HW, Conger SB, Naib Z: Preliminary analysis of oral contraceptive use and risk of developing premalignant lesions of the uterine cervix, in *Pharmacology of Steroid Contraceptive Drugs,* Garratini S, Berendes HW (eds.), New York, Raven, 1977, p. 211.

25. Rinehart W, Felt JC: Debate on oral contraceptives and neoplasia continues: answers remain elusive. Population Reports, Series A, no. 4, 1977.

26. Fuertes de la Haba A, Pelagrainia I, Bangdiwala IS, et al: Changing patterns in cervical cytology among oral and nonoral contraceptive users. J Reprod Med **10**:3, 1973.

27. Berget A, Weber T: Influence of oral contraception on cytology and histology of the cervix uteri: population screening for cervical carcinoma in Maribo Amt 1967–1969. Danish Med Bull **21**:172, 1974.

28. Kirkland JA, Stanley MA: Oral contraceptives and cervical neoplasia. Cancer Cytol **10**:9, 1970.

29. Miller DR: The impact of hormonal contraceptive therapy on a community and effects on cytopathology of the cervix. Amer J Obstet Gynecol **115**:978, 1973.

30. Worth AJ, Boyes DA: A case-control study into the possible effects of birth control pills on pre-clinical carcinoma of the cervix. J Obstet Gynaecol Brit Comm **79**:673, 1972.

31. Thomas DB: Relationship of oral contraceptives to cervical carcinogenesis. Obstet Gynecol **40**:508, 1972.

32. Boyce JG, Lu T, Nelson HJH, et al: Cervical carcinoma and oral contraception. Obstet Gynecol **40**:139, 1972.

33. Melamed MR, Flehinger BJ: Early incidence rates of precancerous cervical lesions in women using oral contraceptives. Gynecol Oncol **1**:290, 1973.

34. Stern E, Forsythe AB, Youkeles L, et al: Steroid contraceptive use and cervical dysplasia; increased risk of progression. Science **196**:1460, 1977.

Oral Contraceptives and Liver Tumors

Paul A. Bloustein, M.D.

A discussion of oral contraceptives and tumors of the liver begins properly with consideration of the effects of contraceptive steroids on hepatic metabolism. That these agents can impair specific hepatic functions became evident shortly after their introduction in 1960. Initially, it was reported that serum transaminase activity and bromsulfophthalein (BSP) retention increased in women given oral contraceptives that contained both an estrogen and a progestogen and that jaundice due to this type of agent could occur (1). In the more than 10 years that have passed since those early reports, the incidence of markedly deranged liver function has diminished as the amount of steroids in oral contraceptives has been reduced. At the same time, additional studies have confirmed that these compounds may alter hepatic functions in the majority of users, although the impairment is rarely so significant as to come to clinical attention.

One of the most sensitive measures of hepatic function is the BSP retention test. Oral contraceptives impair the biliary excretion of anions, as measured by this test, but the effect of this transport interference, while present to some extent in all users of these agents, manifests itself as jaundice in a very small number (2). Liver biopsy in this group shows centrilobular bile stasis with scant inflammation and rare hepatic cell necrosis, and recovery usually occurs within 2 months after withdrawal of the drug (2). Extensive study of this small group of women who develop jaundice while taking oral contraceptives suggests that genetic factors are important in its pathogenesis. Jaundice in this context is seen more frequently in Chile and Scandinavia, countries where cholestasis of pregnancy is also more frequent than in the United States (3). This fact suggests that there is some inherited enzymatic deficiency in these women that becomes overt when the liver is exposed to higher than normal levels of gonadal hormones.

In addition to their effect on BSP retention, oral contraceptives may cause a slight, reversible rise in serum transaminases or alkaline phosphatase in the first few weeks after their introduction (3). In most women, the increase in transaminase activity is transient, suggesting that the hepatocytes are capable of adaptation (1).

It appears that there is no significant difference with respect to their effect on the liver between the two major synthetic estrogens used in oral contraceptives, mestranol and ethynylestradiol (1). What is important is the concentration of the estrogen and the progestogen in the pill, in addition to the structure of the progestogen, the 19-norprogestogens clearly having a more pronounced effect on the liver than the structurally modified progesterones (1).

In addition to the biochemical changes that have just been summarized, ultrastructural alterations have been described in hepatocytes in women on long-term oral contraceptive therapy in the absence of any light microscopic abnormalities (4). The most striking change was an increase in the amount of smooth endoplasmic reticulum. Rather nonspecific mitochondrial abnormalities were also noted. Since the drug-metabolizing enzyme systems of the hepatocyte are located on the smooth endoplasmic reticulum, the increase in the amount of this organelle induced by oral contraceptives probably reflects enzymatic induction by these agents.

While it is relatively easy to describe the metabolic and ultrastructural effects of contraceptive steroids on the liver, it is, with few exceptions, impossible to predict which users of these drugs will develop clinically significant hepatic lesions. Included in this category are cholestasis, peliosis hepatis, and the Budd-Chiari syndrome. In addition to these well-recognized complications of oral contraceptives, the possibility that there may be a causal relationship between such steroids and certain hepatic tumors has generated a great deal of interest and comment. This idea emerged several years ago with the report of Baum et al. (5) and has been strengthened in more recent years by several additional studies (6–10). Two points demonstrated by these studies make the possibility of an etiologic association especially intriguing. These findings are that until the oral contraceptive era, which began in 1960, liver cell adenomas and, to a lesser extent, focal nodular hyperplasia were exceptionally rare lesions (6, 11). Thus Fechner, in a comprehensive review of the literature, could find only eight adequately documented surgical cases of liver cell adenoma prior to 1960 (12). Several other cases had been reported from autopsy series (11). Second, the majority of the more than 100 patients reported in the past several years with benign liver tumors are women in the reproductive years who have used oral contraceptives (10). Thus, prior to the widespread use of contraceptive steroids in this country, hepatocellular adenoma was an exceptionally rare lesion, and the clinical presentation of focal nodular hyperplasia with intralesional hemorrhage and even hepatic rupture was essentially nonexistent. Hepatocellular adenoma is still an uncommon tumor, and catastrophic hemorrhage complicating focal nodular hyperplasia is still a rare event, but both have increased in incidence in recent years, paralleling in some measure the popularity of oral contraceptives.

One of the disturbing features in the welter of reports describing hepatic tumors in women who use birth control pills has been the confused nomenclature that occasionally lumped focal nodular hyperplasia with hepatocellular adenoma without attempting to distinguish between the two. It is absolutely essential to distinguish between these lesions, and hepatocellular carcinoma as well, because all three lesions can occur in women in the child-bearing years. Although they share certain clinical features in common, they are three distinctly different lesions with widely differing implications for the patient.

In late 1973, a liver tumor Registry was established at the University of

Louisville School of Medicine, and data on the first 101 tumors accessioned have recently been published (10). Included were 44 tumors classified as focal nodular hyperplasia, 40 hepatocellular adenomas, 13 hepatocellular carcinomas, and four unclassified tumors thought to be benign. Of the 101 tumors, 81 occurred in oral contraceptive users, and the majority of these women had taken contraceptive steroids for a long time. Of the remaining patients, three were long-term users of estrogens, one patient had a thecoma, six were either pregnant or immediately postpartum, four denied usage of oral contraceptives, and in five the medication history was unknown. The right lobe was involved three times as often as the left, while nine patients had involvement of both lobes. Most of the benign tumors were solitary, but eight patients with hepatocellular adenoma and a like number with focal nodular hyperplasia had multiple tumors.

FOCAL NODULAR HYPERPLASIA

There are several synonyms for this lesion, some of which are listed in Table 1. "Focal cirrhosis" is really a contradiction in terms, because cirrhosis is a widespread process throughout the liver and is not focal. The same objection can be made to the term "lobar cirrhosis." There is nothing pseudo about this lesion—it is a true tumor—and so the term "hepatic pseudotumor" is not appropriate. "Solitary hyperplastic nodule" is not an unsatisfactory term, while some favor "hepatic hamartoma," although others doubt the hamartomatous nature of the lesion. The most popular term at present is focal nodular hyperplasia.

There are several etiologic theories. One holds that this tumor is a hamartoma, by which is meant a disorganized nonneoplastic proliferation of tissues indigenous to an organ. Another popular idea is that this lesion represents a response to local vascular injury. Various vascular lesions are seen in focal nodular hyperplasia, including hypertrophy of arterial walls and inflammation of veins with and without thrombosis. And, in recent years, the idea that this tumor may be secondary to oral contraceptives has been proposed (13), although the evidence of such an association is not as compelling as it is with hepatocellular adenoma (12).

The age range of the 44 women with focal nodular hyperplasia recorded in the liver tumor Registry was 19–46 years, with an average of 29.8 years (10). In general, this tumor is a lesion of women in the child-bearing years, regardless of oral contraceptive use. Vascular lesions were described in focal nodular hyperplasia prior to the introduction of birth control pills and thus cannot be

Table 1. Focal Nodular Hyperplasia: Synonyms

Focal cirrhosis
Lobar cirrhosis
Hepatic pseudotumor
Solitary hyperplastic nodule
Hepatic hamartoma
Nodular transformation

ascribed to the use of these agents (12). What might be related to oral contraceptives is hemorrhage within a preexisting lesion of focal nodular hyperplasia, because only since the advent of the oral contraceptive era have patients with this lesion presented with significant intrahepatic hemorrhage or actual hepatic rupture (12).

The majority of patients with focal nodular hyperplasia unrelated to contraceptive steroid use are asymptomatic. This may also be true for those lesions that occur in women on oral contraceptives. Liver function tests are generally within normal limits. Since the majority of these lesions are asymptomatic and are usually discovered incidentally during the course of unrelated surgery, there is some question as to whether these lesions require resection. There is evidence that they may decrease in size (10, 14), and therefore a rational approach to a woman taking oral contraceptives who has focal nodular hyperplasia that has not hemorrhaged would be discontinuation of the medication.

One very rare complication of focal nodular hyperplasia is the development of hepatocellular carcinoma within a portion of the lesion. This phenomenon has been well documented in one case (10) and reported in a second case (15), although review of the latter report leaves some doubt as to the nature of the benign tumor from which the hepatocellular carcinoma arose.

Since the majority of these lesions are asymptomatic and are discovered incidentally or at autopsy, it is almost impossible to determine the exact incidence of focal nodular hyperplasia in the population. It is equally as difficult to determine whether oral contraceptives have had any effect on the incidence of the lesion, but, as Fechner has indicated, there is no convincing evidence of an etiologic association (12).

HEPATOCELLULAR ADENOMA

As indicated above, hepatocellular adenoma was an exceptionally uncommon tumor prior to the widespread use of oral contraceptives. However, in the past 4 years alone, 40 of these tumors have been accessioned in the liver tumor Registry (10). The majority of these patients have been women in the child-bearing years (age range, 14–47 years; average, 29.5 years). While hepatocellular adenoma can occur in women not taking contraceptive steroids and with no endogenous hormonal abnormalities, and has been seen rarely in infants and men, the majority of the patients reported in recent years have been users of oral contraceptives. Some of the contraceptive agents that have been associated with liver cell adenomas are listed in Table 2. They include many of the commonly

Table 2.   Drugs Associated With Adenomas

Enovid (norethynodrel and mestranol)
Norinyl (norethindrone and mestranol)
Ortho-Novum (norethindrone and mestranol)
Ovulen (ethynodiol and mestranol)
Oracon (dimethisterone and ethynylestradiol)
Ovral (norgestrel and ethynylestradiol)

used preparations. The usual duration of usage of these drugs at the time of presentation of a patient with an adenoma is on the order of several years. Patients have been seen, however, who had no more than 6 months of exposure. As pointed out by Edmondson et al. (7), the risk increases dramatically with duration of use, especially after 5 years.

There are various patterns of clinical presentation. The majority of patients either have a palpable mass with or without right upper quadrant discomfort or develop symptoms after hemorrhage into the tumor or actual hepatic rupture. Only a small number of these tumors are discovered during the course of unrelated surgery.

The liver function studies are usually normal. α-Fetoprotein, when measured, has been normal. Barium studies of the upper gastrointestinal tract may show displacement of viscera by the tumor, and liver scan may show a mass, but these findings are of little discriminatory aid in the differential diagnosis. Some feel that hepatic arteriography can distinguish between benign and malignant hepatic tumors (5) and can distinguish metastatic tumors from primary growths (6). Percutaneous needle biopsy is generally felt to be contraindicated because of the risk of hemorrhage from these usually very vascular tumors.

The major complications of hepatocellular adenoma include hemorrhage into the tumor, presenting as the sudden onset of abdominal pain, and hemoperitoneum following rupture of the tumor through Glisson's capsule. As is true with focal nodular hyperplasia, the risk of hemorrhage and rupture with liver cell adenoma is magnified considerably when the patient is using oral contraceptives (12). Some have suggested in the past that hepatocellular adenoma may undergo malignant transformation (16) or "shade imperceptibly into carcinoma" (17), but this contention has never been substantiated conclusively. The possibility of production of biologically active substances by the tumor is an intriguing idea and, while not proven, is suggested by the following case report:

> A female in her early twenties was seen by a physician for investigation of intractable diarrhea. A right upper quadrant mass was palpated and the patient underwent abdominal exploration. A large tumor of the right lobe of the liver was found and the patient was referred to the University of Colorado Medical Center for definitive surgery. A trisegmentectomy was performed with removal of a large hepatocellular adenoma in excess of 2000 gm. The diarrhea resolved following resection of the tumor. Assays of both serum and tumor for a prostaglandin thought to increase intestinal motility were negative.

One other case in the literature was quite similar (11). These authors reported a 22-year-old woman with 6 months of diarrhea, rectal bleeding, and lower abdominal pain. Barium enema revealed mucosal ulcerations in the ascending colon. Workup for pathogens was negative. The diarrhea cleared following incomplete resection of a very large hepatocellular adenoma. Unfortunately, the tumor tissue was not further studied. Did the tumor secrete a substance that caused the diarrhea directly or, perhaps, secondarily through the induction of a focal colitis?

The natural history of these tumors is somewhat variable. The possibility of intralesional hemorrhage with or without rupture of the liver has already been mentioned. The most exciting possibility appears to be the chance of regression of the tumor after withdrawal of the contraceptive agent. Several such cases have been reported (6, 9, 18, 19) and serve to suggest an alternative to surgery in certain situations. However, it must be remembered that cessation of contraceptive steroid therapy does not fully remove the risk of hemorrhage from an adenoma (12). Can these tumors achieve a certain size and then stabilize and remain asymptomatic for years in the face of continued contraceptive hormone use? The answer is not known.

HEPATOCELLULAR CARCINOMA

Liver cell carcinoma has been reported in women using contraceptive steroids (10) and estrogen-like drugs (20), but the number of such cases in no way represents the type of increase in frequency that has been seen with hepatocellular adenoma. These few cases of hepatocellular carcinoma may bear no etiologic relationship to oral contraceptive use, although conclusive judgment on this possibility must be reserved pending the publication of more data.

Do oral contraceptives cause liver tumors? As discussed above, there is no convincing evidence that the incidence of focal nodular hyperplasia or hepatocellular carcinoma has increased since the introduction of these drugs. As Fechner pointed out (12), what has changed somewhat is the mode of clinical presentation of focal nodular hyperplasia in some women on oral contraceptives. However, a definitive judgment on this question must be kept in abeyance until more data, both clinical and experimental, have been studied.

A much stronger argument can be made with respect to the etiologic association between contraceptive steroids and hepatocellular adenoma. It begins with the striking increase in incidence of this rare tumor in recent years, the majority occurring in women using oral contraceptives. And it is buttressed by the fact that a variety of liver tumors have been reported in people receiving other steroid hormones. Thus, liver cell carcinomas have been reported in patients on long-term androgenic anabolic steroid therapy given for a variety of reasons, including aplastic anemia, Fanconi's anemia, paroxysmal nocturnal hemoglobinuria, hypopituitarism, and cryptorchidism (21–24). While most of these tumors have remained confined to the liver and several have regressed after withdrawal of androgen therapy (22, 24), at least one has metastasized (24). In addition, hepatoblastoma has been seen in a woman taking oral contraceptives (25), and several hepatocellular adenomas have been reported in patients on androgenic anabolic steroids (24, 26, 27). Certainly, the occurrence of some of these tumors in patients on steroid hormone therapy may be coincidental, but to regard all of them in that light without further investigation, data collection, and experimentation courts the danger of missing what could be a significant association.

Assuming that oral contraceptives are etiologically related to hepatocellular adenoma and, perhaps, to other liver tumors, which component of the compound is responsible for the tumor? Or do both components, the synthetic estrogen and progestogen, play a role? The answer is unknown. Some feel that estrogens are probably the predominant factor, because tumors have been seen in women taking conjugated equine estrogens, in women in late pregnancy or the early postpartum period, and even in a woman with a feminizing ovarian tumor (28). In addition, estrogens have been associated with tumor production in other tissues, and small doses of estrogens can promote liver regeneration in rats (1). On the other hand, progestogens are structurally related to the androgenic anabolic steroids (1), and, as mentioned in the preceding paragraph, both liver cell carcinomas and adenomas have been seen in patients receiving the latter agents. The increase of smooth endoplasmic reticulum in hepatocytes of women taking oral contraceptives has been attributed to the progestogenic component (1), and this phenomenon is the morphologic counterpart of enzymatic induction. It is known that some substances require metabolic conversion by hepatic enzymes before they can exercise their neoplastic effect, and perhaps the enzymatic induction produced by progestogens plays a role in such conversion (29).

Obviously, the final answer regarding the relationship between oral contraceptives and liver tumors is not known. However, a fairly strong, albeit somewhat circumstantial, case has been made to support the idea that contraceptive steroids may be associated etiologically with hepatocellular adenoma and may play a role in the hemorrhagic complications of focal nodular hyperplasia. As more data are collected, this complex and confusing relationship should be further clarified.

REFERENCES

1. Adlercreutz H, Tenhunen R: Some aspects of the interaction between natural and synthetic female sex hormones and the liver. Amer J Med **49**:630, 1970.

2. Weindling H, Henry JB: Laboratory test results altered by "the pill." J Amer Med Ass **229**:1762, 1974.

3. Oral contraceptives and the liver. Brit Med J **4**:430, 1974.

4. Perez V, Gorosdisch S, DeMartire J, et al: Oral contraceptives: long-term use produces fine structural changes in liver mitochondria. Science **165**:805, 1969.

5. Baum JK, Holtz F, Bookstein JJ, et al: Possible association between benign hepatomas and oral contraceptives. Lancet **2**:926, 1973.

6. Ameriks JA, Thompson NW, Frey CF, et al: Hepatic cell adenomas, spontaneous liver rupture, and oral contraceptives. Arch Surg **110**:548, 1975.

7. Edmondson HA, Henderson B, Benton B: Liver-cell adenomas associated with use of oral contraceptives. N Engl J Med **294**:470, 1976.

8. McAvoy JM, Tompkins RK, Longmire WP Jr: Benign hepatic tumors and their association with oral contraceptives. Arch Surg **111**:761, 1976.

9. Nissen ED, Kent DR, Nissen SE, et al: Association of liver tumors with oral contraceptives. Obstet Gynecol **48**:49, 1976.

10. Christopherson WM, Mays ET, Barrows G: A clinicopathologic study of steroid-related liver tumors. Amer J Surg Pathol **1**:31, 1977.

11. Albritton DR, Tompkins RK, Longmire WP Jr: Hepatic cell adenoma: a report of four cases. Ann Surg **180**:14, 1974.

12. Fechner RE: Benign hepatic lesions and orally administered contraceptives. Human Pathol **8**:255, 1977.

13. Mays ET, Christopherson WM, Barrows GH: Focal nodular hyperplasia of the liver. Possible relationship to oral contraceptives. Amer J Clin Pathol **61**:735, 1974.

14. Ross D, Pina J, Mirza M, et al: Regression of focal nodular hyperplasia after discontinuation of oral contraceptives. Ann Intern Med **85:**203, 1976.

15. Davis M, Portmann B, Searle M, et al: Histological evidence of carcinoma in a hepatic tumor associated with oral contraceptives. Brit Med J **4:**496, 1975.

16. Edmondson HA: Tumors of the liver and intrahepatic bile ducts, *Atlas of Tumor Pathology*, Washington, DC, Armed Forces Institute of Pathology, 1958, section VII, fascicle 25.

17. Ackerman LV: *Surgical Pathology*, St. Louis, CV Mosby, 1964.

18. Edmondson HA, Reynolds TB, Henderson B, et al: Regression of liver cell adenomas associated with oral contraceptives. Ann Intern Med **86:**180, 1977.

19. Cornish PG III: Liver cell adenoma (Letter to the Editor). J Amer Med Ass **235:**249, 1976.

20. Thalassinos NC, Lymberatos C, Hadjioannou J, et al: Liver-cell carcinoma after long-term estrogen-like drugs. Lancet **1:**270, 1974.

21. Bernstein MS, Hunter RL, Yachnin S: Hepatoma and peliosis hepatis developing in a patient with Fanconi's anemia. N Engl J Med **284:**1135, 1971.

22. Johnson FL, Feagler JR, Lerner KG, et al: Association of androgenic-anabolic steroid therapy with development of hepatocellular carcinoma. Lancet **2:**1273, 1972.

23. Meadows AT, Naiman JL, Valdes-Dapena M: Hepatoma associated with androgen therapy for aplastic anemia. J Pediat **84:**109, 1974.

24. Farrell GC, Joshua DE, Uren RF, et al: Androgen-induced hepatoma. Lancet **1:**430, 1975.

25. Meyer P, LiVolsi VA, Cornog JL: Hepatoblastoma associated with an oral contraceptive. Lancet **2:**1387, 1974.

26. Bruguera M: Letter to the Editor. Lancet **1:**1295, 1975.

27. Sweeney EC, Evans DJ: Hepatic lesions in patients treated with synthetic anabolic steroids. J Clin Pathol **29:**626, 1976.

28. Christopherson WM, Mays ET: Liver tumors and contraceptive steroids: experience with the first one hundred registry patients. J Nat Cancer Inst **58:**167, 1977.

29. Lingeman CH: Liver-cell neoplasms and oral contraceptives. Lancet **1:**64, 1974.

Pathologic Aspects of Tumors and Tumor-like Lesions in Women Taking Oral Contraceptive Hormones

Robert E. Fechner, M.D.

LIVER TUMORS

A critical analysis of the Anglo-American literature on benign hepatic tumors between 1940 and 1976 has been published recently (1). It provides a group of cases seen before 1960, when hormones were approved by the Federal Drug Administration for use as oral contraceptives. Women with liver tumors reported since 1960 may have been taking contraceptive steroids whether or not it is specifically stated in the history. Cases published prior to 1960 are valuable because they form a control group for comparison of either clinical or pathologic aspects of lesions removed from users of hormones.

A second notable date is 1973, when the possible relation of oral contraceptives to liver tumors was raised (2). The literature on liver tumors since 1973 has dealt almost exclusively with women taking hormones. It appears that the primary consideration for publication is that the patient be taking contraceptive steroids, a factor that has resulted in a strong correlation between liver tumors and hormones. Anecdotal literature can provide new information, but it can also become disproportionately weighted toward a positive association between the two selected events. Proper perspective can be attained only by utilizing appropriate controls or by the reporting of consecutive cases of tumors from patients who are unselected in regard to contraceptive modality.

Since 1973, there have been approximately 300 instances of benign liver tumors reported from women taking contraceptive hormones (3–21). Other women with liver tumors published since 1960 have had a history of oral contraceptive usage obtained in retrospect (22–29). Pathologists have not actively participated in many papers, and the gross and microscopic pathologic

111

data have been meager. A few patients have been included in two or more reports. In one paper, a given lesion is diagnosed as focal nodular hyperplasia, and in another paper, the identical lesion is called liver cell adenoma (26, 30–32). One "Registry" has ignored histologic distinctions altogether (33).

The confusion has been reflected by the many diagnostic terms given to the benign tumors from women taking contraceptive hormones. They have been labeled focal nodular hyperplasia, hamartoma, adenoma, benign hepatoma, minimal deviation hepatoma, and adenoma with focal nodular hyperplasia. In the cases where adequate descriptions or illustrations are given, it is obvious that many of the seemingly disparate diagnostic terms are being applied to lesions that are fully characteristic of either focal nodular hyperplasia or liver cell adenoma, which were clearly separated and defined by Edmondson in the late 1950s (34). The gross and microscopic criteria are sharp and have continued to be used by Edmondson and other authorities to the present time (35–38). The distinction between these tumors is more important than classification merely for the sake of classification. The risk for potentially fatal hemorrhage differs markedly between the two lesions, and proper diagnosis can influence the clinical management.

The criteria for the diagnosis of focal nodular hyperplasia are one or more grossly visible nodules in an otherwise normal liver, a predominance of normal hepatic cells, bile ductules or small bile ducts, and fibrous septa, which almost always radiate from a broad central fibrous zone (Figure 1). In addition, there is often a dense inflammatory infiltrate in some of the septa. This infiltrate consists mainly of lymphocytes but is not a criterion for diagnosis.

Liver cell adenoma is a tumor that is composed of hepatocytes with nuclear variation no greater than that seen in normal liver and of Kupffer cells. Liver cell adenoma, by definition, does not contain bile ducts or ductules. It may contain bile in canaliculi, but cholangioles are never formed. Focal nodular hyperplasia and liver cell adenoma defined by Edmondson's criteria are mutually exclusive

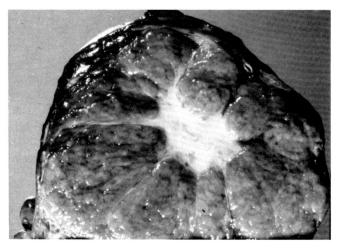

Figure 1. Cut surface of focal nodular hyperplasia has coarse nodules of hepatic parenchyma separated by thin fibrous septa that radiate from central fibrous area. The mass is 7 cm wide. Patient had taken oral contraceptives for 3 years.

diagnoses. The crucial difference is the presence of bile ducts in nodular hyperplasia and their total absence in adenomas. It is important to realize that the ductules in nodular hyperplasia are concentrated at the edges of nodules and not widely intermixed with the liver cells. Furthermore, distribution of bile ductules is uneven, and large blocks of tissue may contain none. For example, Christopherson et al. found ductules in only two of 17 blocks in one case of nodular hyperplasia (20).

Turning to the surgical literature prior to 1960, we identified 13 adults with well-documented focal nodular hyperplasia (1). Ten were women who were 23, 28 (three women), 32, 38, 39, 46, 47, and 63 years old. Since 1960, 26 fully documented cases of focal nodular hyperplasia have been reported in small series exclusive of those in Christopherson's Registry. Twenty-three of these 26 cases were women 21–51 years of age, 13 of whom were between 21 and 29 years old. Therefore, the age range before and after the oral contraceptive era is virtually identical, with approximately half of the patients being in the third decade of life regardless of whether they were taking hormones.

We have compared our cases of focal nodular hyperplasia from hormone users with lesions removed from patients who had never used hormones. The gross and microscopic features have not differed. Furthermore, a comparison of descriptions from the pre-1960 literature shows no difference.

In other series, however, there is an important change in a few cases reported since 1960. Prior to 1960, no case of nodular hyperplasia had ever been reported that presented with life-threatening hemorrhage, although small foci of old or recent hemorrhage could be found in surgically resected lesions (39). In 1967, a 25-year-old woman was reported who had hemorrhage from nodular hyperplasia, but there is no information regarding oral contraceptive usage (40). Since that time, six cases of well-documented hyperplasia have presented with intrahepatic or intraperitoneal bleeding (41). It must be noted at this point that one recent series stated to be nodular hyperplasia with hemorrhage lacks both descriptive and photographic proof that the lesions are hyperplasia. They more likely represent adenomas (42).

The only pathologic difference between lesions removed from women taking hormones and those from nonhormone users is the presence of hemorrhagic necrosis. Mays et al. have described a variety of abnormalities in the lesions that have bled (18). These abnormalities include arterial medial hypertrophy with varying degrees of occlusion, phlebitis, organizing thrombi, and intimal proliferation in small vessels. These investigators felt that the changes might have caused the necrosis but were aware that they could be merely secondary to the necrosis. Similar vascular alterations have been described in other cases of nodular hyperplasia from women taking hormones in whom hemorrhage was absent (Figure 2) (17, 19). Markedly abnormal vessels can exist without producing bleeding and, therefore, are not secondary to hemorrhage in these particular instances. Furthermore, arterial and venous hypertrophy were described by Edmondson in 1958 (34) and by Benz and Baggenstoss (43), who found "occasional venous thrombi" in lesions of noninfarcted nodular hyperplasia in autopsy material before the contraceptive era began. We have also seen medial hypertrophy and intimal thickening in hyperplasia from women who had an unequivocally negative history of hormone usage. For these reasons, one should not too quickly attribute the vascular changes to hormones. Nonetheless, it is

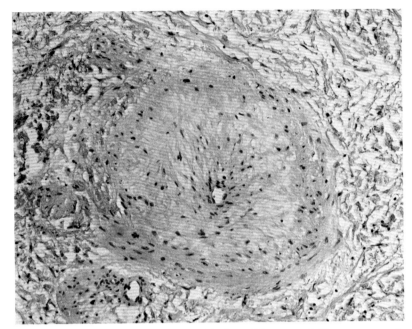

Figure 2. Almost total occlusion of vessel is found in central fibrous area of nodular hyperplasia. No hemorrhage was present.

quite possible that there is a quantitative increase in vascular changes in women taking oral contraceptives that is secondary to hormone usage. Even more likely, some of these women are probably susceptible to thrombotic episodes that result in occlusion sufficient to produce necrosis and subsequent hemorrhage.

It is appropriate at this point to acknowledge that hepatic venoocclusive disease has been reported in approximately a dozen women taking oral contraceptives who had no tumors. Most cases have involved thrombosis of major hepatic veins, but in one patient, sublobular and central veins were involved with an intimal proliferation in addition to thrombi (44).

In tabulating individual reports, focal nodular hyperplasia has been distributed evenly between the left and right lobes both before and after 1960, including patients taking oral contraceptives (1), with the exception of the series of Christopherson et al. (20). These workers have found the right lobe to be involved three times more often than the left. The frequency of multiple lesions, about 15%, is similar before and after 1960 (1). In an autopsy series studied before the hormone era (43), five of 34 cases of nodular hyperplasia had multiple nodules, a figure similar to the frequency in the recently reported surgical series. One remarkable case bears emphasis. Mays et al. reported a second lesion of nodular hyperplasia in a woman who continued to use oral contraceptives after the first resection (45).

In addition to the above alterations, less dramatic changes are found in the noninfarcted parenchyma. Dilated sinusoids are present focally, which may be sufficiently broad and confluent to form small lakes of blood without apparent necrosis of hepatocytes (Figure 3). We have seen one example of sinusoidal dilatation in the adjacent liver (Figure 4). Similar foci of sinusoidal dilatation

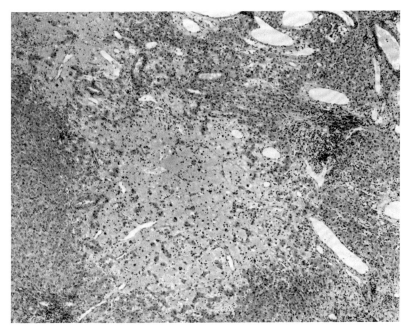

Figure 3. Irregular distribution of vessels in peripheral area of focal nodular hyperplasia. Replacement of parenchyma by blood is seen centrally, with a few hepatocytes remaining. Same case as that in Figures 1 and 2.

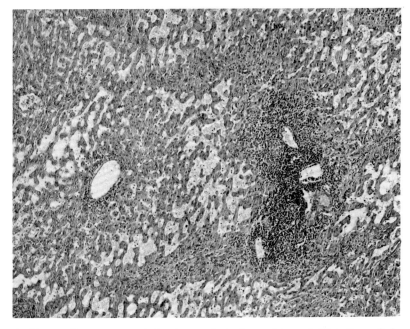

Figure 4. Liver adjacent to nodular hyperplasia has midzonal dilatation of sinusoids. Portal area (*right*) is accentuated by lymphocytic infiltrate that has no recognized relation to hormonal usage.

have also been described in needle biopsies from patients without tumor masses in which the sinusoidal dilatation has been periportal (46).

LIVER CELL ADENOMA

Liver cell adenomas were extremely rare lesions before 1960, and we have accepted only eight cases as being adequately documented (1). Since 1960, seven of 10 women with adenomas who are known to have never used hormones were between the ages of 19 and 27 (1). As with nodular hyperplasia, young women are those most likely to develop liver cell adenomas, even if they are not taking hormones.

Multiple adenomas were reported in eight of 40 patients by Christopherson et al. (20). In a compilation of smaller series, nine of 36 women reported since 1960 have had multiple adenomas. Three of the cases occurred in women using hormones, but four of seven women with a definitely negative history for oral contraceptives also had multiple lesions (1).

Liver cell adenomas are sharply circumscribed but may or may not have a grossly visible thin capsule (Figure 5). The intact adenoma varies in color from light tan to yellow. It may be homogeneous or have a faint nodularity, with the nodules varying from a few millimeters to 1 cm in size. The coarse, bulging nodularity of focal nodular hyperplasia is not seen because the nodules of adenoma are not demarcated by fibrous septa.

Adenomas that have presented with clinical signs of hemorrhage are usually almost totally replaced with blood (Figure 6). Irregular islands of tumor may be

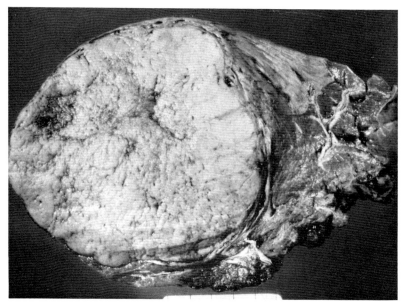

Figure 5. Liver cell adenoma has pale yellow color, in contrast with normal liver (*right*). Mass is 11 cm in diameter, with finely granular cut surface. Patient had taken oral contraceptives for 5 years and presented with palpable mass.

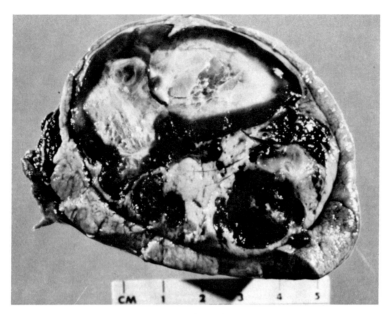

Figure 6. Liver cell adenoma with hemorrhage into the tumor. Patient had taken oral contraceptives for 5 years and presented with acute pain.

scattered within the hemorrhagic tissue. In some instances, the massive hemorrhage leaves virtually no recognizable neoplasm. Only a tiny rim of yellow tissue 2–4 mm wide persists at the periphery (Figure 7). It is likely that cases of hepatic rupture in which only a hematoma was found may be adenomas totally destroyed by the bleeding (47).

The small adenomas are especially likely to be unencapsulated, whereas larger

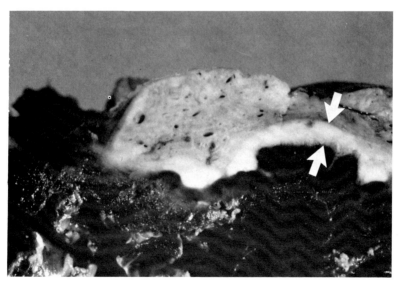

Figure 7. Liver cell adenoma almost totally replaced by hemorrhage. The only remnants of tumor were a bright yellow rim 2–3 mm wide (distance between arrows) that persisted at edge of tumor. The lesion is sharply demarcated but without grossly visible capsule.

tumors have a thin capsule (Figure 8). Edmondson et al. note that one case with multiple small adenomas showed continuity of the cells of the tumor nodules with the normal hepatocytes (48). They point out that adenomas associated with hormones may arise by transformation of multiple normal cells, which then become autonomous, with development of their own blood supply and secondary encapsulation. Arteriographic studies have shown newly formed peripheral feeding vessels around the edge of large adenomas, an appearance that contrasts with the arteriographic pattern of focal nodular hyperplasia (49).

The histologic appearance of adenomas is diverse. The simplest form is the arrangement of cells in cords one or two cells thick, closely resembling normal liver (Figure 9). The hepatocytes are lined by Kupffer cells. More often, the hepatocytes are in a patternless sheet, and the nuclei of Kupffer cells are barely discernible. On occasion, acini are found (Figure 10).

The individual cells may have finely granular eosinophilic cytoplasm indistinguishable from that of normal hepatocytes. More commonly, the cells are slightly larger and more polyhedral. The cytoplasm is less dense because it is frequently rich in glycogen, and accumulations are almost always far more abundant than in the adjacent liver. On rare occasions, vacuoles of fat have distended the cells of the adenoma. Bile is uncommonly identifiable, but small bile plugs were illustrated in one case (20), and bile was seen in canaliculi in another case (50). It is again emphasized that bile ductules or cholangioles are not present in adenomas.

Dilated sinusoids and irregular blood lakes may form, even in the absence of hemorrhage (51). The distribution of vessels within adenomas appears to be

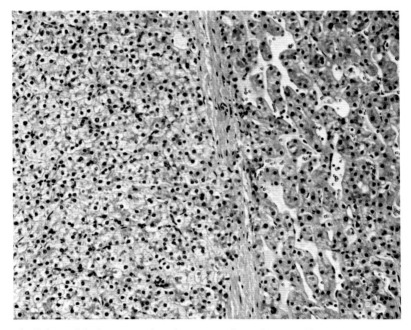

Figure 8. Edge of lesion seen in Figure 4. Discontinuous fibrous capsule separates adenoma (*left*) from normal liver (*right*). Hepatocytes in the tumor are more lightly staining due to large amounts of glycogen.

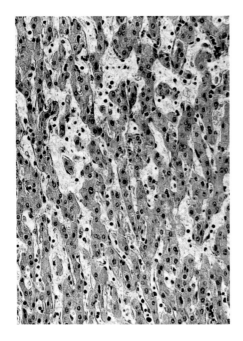

Figure 9. Trabecular pattern of liver cell adenoma with normal-appearing hepatocytes. Distended sinusoids are conspicuous.

random, with areas of numerous vessels alternating with broad zones that lack vessels. Most of the vascular channels are thin-walled, but in one case, intimal thickening is seen in the photograph of an adenoma although not discussed in the text (52).

The nuclear variation in the hepatocytes of adenomas is considerable. In general, nuclei are of about the same size and chromatin density as those of

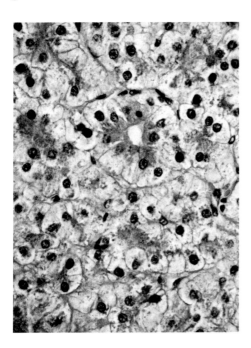

Figure 10. Liver cell adenoma with closely packed polyhedral cells occasionally forming acini. Abundant glycogen was present.

normal hepatocytes. They may, however, range up to four or five times the normal diameter and assume a more vesicular appearance, with clumping of chromatin along the nuclear membrane. All gradations of both size and density of nuclear staining are present between these extremes. Binucleated cells are common, and cells with three to five or more nuclei may occur. Mitotic figures have not been described in adenomas. The great frequency of binucleated cells is ample evidence of cellular replication and is the expected indicator of growth for nonmalignant proliferation of hepatocytes.

The regression of both focal nodular hyperplasia (53) and liver cell adenomas (47, 54) has been reported after these women stopped taking hormones. How much of this regression is the result of shrinkage of the tumor mass and how much is the consequence of resolution of the hematoma is difficult to determine in some cases. It must be emphasized that cessation of hormone usage does not assure that a lesion will regress or not hemorrhage. Two women who had discontinued hormone usage and completed a subsequent pregnancy ruptured an adenoma at 9 days and 5 weeks postpartum, respectively (15, 50). Another woman who had stopped taking hormones 9 months previously went into shock from hemorrhage into an adenoma (11).

Brander et al. have described a unique case of diffuse hyperplasia of the liver in a 24-year-old woman. For 4 years, she had taken hormones at doses four times greater than the oral contraceptive dose because of irregular vaginal bleeding. She died of hepatic rupture, and unencapsulated tumors ranging from 0.2 to 6 cm were present in both lobes. In addition, there were microscopic nodules of hepatocytes (55).

Ultrastructural studies on the livers of women taking oral contraceptives have shown alterations of ergastoplasm and mitochondria. Nonneoplastic liver cells from women taking hormones have demonstrated dilatation and vesicle formation in both the smooth and rough profiles of the ergastoplasm (56). This finding could reflect induction and/or activation of microsomal drug-metabolizing enzymes, which are responsible for the metabolism of at least some synthetic and endogenous sex steroids.

By contrast, Kay and Schatzki found no conspicuous alteration in the ergastoplasm (ER) of a liver cell adenoma from women taking hormones (22, 23), and Horvath et al. noted specifically that the ER in their adenoma did not differ from normal hepatocytes "in any way" (3). On the other hand, in one extensive study of liver cell adenomas, smooth ER was consistently decreased, but no drug histories are given (57). The decrease of ER in these lesions may be analogous to experimentally induced minimal deviation hepatomas, which have a decreased activity of microsomal enzymes when compared to normal (58).

The mitochondrial alterations in both nonneoplastic and neoplastic hepatocytes consist of mitochondriomegaly, with formation of intramitochondrial crystalloid inclusions (Figure 11). The inclusions have been the focus of considerable attention, but their pathogenesis and chemical structure remain obscure. They are seen in livers injured through such diverse insults as obstructive jaundice, alcohol, viral hepatitis, obesity, and toxic hepatitis (59). Gonzales-Angulo et al. found inclusions in livers during pregnancy but not in women whose pregnancy had terminated 5–12 months before the biopsy, and they suggested that the inclusions are a reflection of increased metabolic demand (56). Perez et al. found

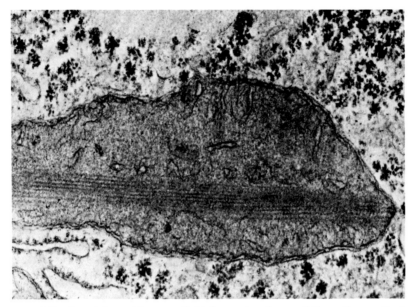

Figure 11. Mitochondrion with crystalloid formation in a cell from liver cell adenoma. Adjacent cytoplasm contains glycogen. Patient had taken oral contraceptives for 5 years.

inclusions in eight of 13 women receiving hormones for more than 1 year (60). There was no correlation with the duration of therapy, because one patient taking hormones for 30 months had no inclusions, whereas they were numerous in two women after only 1 year of treatment. The presence of inclusions did not correlate with abnormal liver function tests. After discontinuance of hormones for 6 months, repeat biopsies in six women contained diminished numbers of persistent inclusions (61). Identical inclusions have also been illustrated in the two liver cell adenomas mentioned above (3, 22), but the significance of the inclusions in both neoplastic and nonneoplastic liver cells is difficult to assess because of the inconsistency of ultrastructural studies on apparently normal liver. Bhagwat et al. examined livers from five persons (one female) defined as normal by the absence of a history for liver disease, normal hepatic function tests, and a grossly and microscopically normal liver (62). None contained inclusions. Using similar criteria of normalcy, others have found inclusions in 15 of 18 livers, but neither the sex nor a statement regarding drug therapy is given in these reports (63–65). Whatever the mechanism for their formation, the inclusions in patients taking oral contraception seem to be, at best, a quantitative and not a qualitative difference when compared with normal liver or liver damaged by other agents.

Hepatocellular carcinoma has been reported in several women taking oral contraceptive hormones. One of the earliest reports (66) has subsequently had the pathologic diagnoses revised to adenoma, and the women are well (67). Galloway et al. have used the term "minimal deviation hepatoma" for two tumors, but it seems likely that their lesions are within the realm of adenoma (16). The report by Davis et al. illustrates widespread bizarre cytologic alterations of sufficient degree to warrant the diagnosis of hepatoma on histologic grounds, but no follow-up report is available (68). One case of mixed bile duct carcinoma and hepatoma has been briefly reported (69). The best documented hepatomas are the 13 reported by Christopherson et al., who have illustrated venous invasion and described distant metastases in some cases (20, 45). The cytologic features are those of malignancy, with bizarre nuclei and abnormal mitotic figures. Eosinophilic globular cytoplasmic inclusions were present in a few instances and, ultrastructurally, consisted of dense filamentous material with the appearance reported previously in hepatomas, including some from males (20).

One remarkable case suggests the origin of a hepatoma in a tumor mass that also had the characteristics of focal nodular hyperplasia (20). This is a unique case and should be viewed as a curiosity and not influence the management of otherwise typical lesions of nodular hyperplasia. There is no reason that the hepatocytes in nodular hyperplasia should be immune from malignant transformation, but if this phenomenon occurs, it is an extraordinarily rare event. The possibility of a collision phenomenon is an alternative explanation for the above case. In other series of nodular hyperplasia in which the lesion was confirmed by biopsy but not resected, there has been no evidence of subsequent neoplasm (70). Furthermore, the 38 patients reported in autopsy series carried their tumors to the end of life without adverse effects (43, 71).

One other malignant neoplasm, a hepatoblastoma, has been reported in a 19-year-old girl taking oral contraceptives (72). This case is intriguing, because hepatoblastoma is usually found in infants, and the cases described in adults have all been in males (73). Nonetheless, no cause and effect relation can be implied on the basis of a single patient.

The role of hormones in the malignant tumors of the liver must be viewed with caution. Hepatocellular carcinoma occurs frequently in young adults, and in older people, a distribution that preceded the hormone era (74). A search of one large Registry of hormone users has yielded no cases of hepatic tumors in 116,000 women-years of exposure (75). Furthermore, the advent of many other new drugs over the last two decades must be kept in mind. It is easy to ask for a history of hormone therapy and, having obtained an affirmative statement, to assume that it is a contributing factor. Equal attention, however, should be directed to other drugs that can alter metabolism and morphology of hepatocytes, such as barbiturates and diazepam (Valium) (76). With many millions of women exposed to oral contraceptives in the United States alone, every disease can be expected by pure chance within such a large population. This is especially true for benign liver tumors, in which the peak years for their "spontaneous" occurrence are the same as the peak years that women take contraceptive hormones.

CERVIX

The exocervix has not been found to undergo unusual cytologic or histologic alterations of the type found in the endocervix or endometrium. Studies dealing with the relation of oral contraceptives to preneoplastic or neoplastic conditions of the cervix have, therefore, been epidemiologic and are discussed elsewhere in this volume. One interesting idea for the pathogenesis of dysplasia in some women taking hormones was suggested by Whitehead et al. based on cytologic observations (77). Squamous cells with atypical large nuclei reminded them of megaloblastic changes found in other cells in certain vitamin deficiencies. Despite the fact that the pretreatment levels of folic acid were normal in their patients with dysplasia, a 3-week course of folic acid therapy resulted in conversion of the cervical epithelium to a normal appearance. They hypothesized that oral contraceptives may have resulted in a localized interference of folic acid metabolism at the end-organ level. In another study, oral contraceptives had no apparent effect in two women with metastatic squamous carcinoma (78).

In contrast to the exocervix, the endocervix is extremely responsive to oral contraceptives in some women. It can exhibit an increase in the size of the columnar epithelium, hypersecretion, increased vascularity, stromal edema, and pseudodecidual stromal reaction (79, 80). These changes will regress 2–3 months after cessation of medication (81). The hormones alter the cervical mucus, decreasing sperm penetrability (82), prevent crystallization (83), and modify the normal protein components (84). Sequential agents have a less profound effect but also will produce an abnormal cumulative increase in acid mucosubstance after repeated cycles of therapy (85). The cervical mucus has slightly different qualities, depending on the drug used (86), suggesting that, in addition to pituitary inhibition by oral contraceptives, there is a direct effect on the glands, at least by some hormones (87).

From the pathologist's viewpoint, the most important alteration in the endocervix is microglandular hyperplasia, which can be mistaken for adenocarcinoma. This condition was first described in 1967 (88), and several subsequent reports have confirmed the association (89–91). Although it was initially thought that microglandular hyperplasia was pathognomonic for hormone usage, many additional cases have been described from women who have never used hormones, including pregnant women (92). In the latter patients, the lesions have sometimes been polypoid masses clinically identical to some of the large lesions described in users of hormones.

The frequency of microglandular hyperplasia has ranged from less than 2% (93) to 44% (94) of cervices examined after conization. The high frequency in the latter series is explained by the fact that the cases were minutely studied, and areas that measured only 1 or 2 mm in size were counted. Using this level of sensitivity, 11% of nonusers of hormones also showed hyperplasia in this study.

Microglandular hyperplasia may last up to 1 year after the use of hormones has been discontinued (92). Therefore, glandular proliferation, once initiated, may persist for a considerable time without requiring continuing exogenous hormone support. This situation contrasts with that of the endometrium, which will revert to normal within two or three cycles after therapy has been terminated. In hormone users, approximately half of the lesions have been discovered on routine examination of asymptomatic women. Another one fourth of women have complained of postcoital bleeding or spotting, and the remaining patients have had vaginal discharge. Most women have been in their 20s or 30s, although one patient under therapy for endometrial adenocarcinoma was 66 years old (90). Clinically, the cervix may appear normal but more typically shows erosion, friable polypoid excrescences, a single endocervical polyp, or diffuse enlargement.

On cytologic examination, women using hormones may shed broad sheets of columnar cells, including multinucleated forms with enlarged nuclei (95). Mildly abnormal squamous cells of the type seen in squamous metaplasia or the nonspecific alterations of chronic cervicitis have also been reported (96).

Microscopically, the major site of activity is in the superficial portion of the endocervical mucosa, resulting in the exophytic lesions that are clinically visible (Figure 12). In rare cases, there may be partial involvement of a deeper gland by intraluminal proliferation of small glands similar to the process on the surface (94, 96). In either site, the process results in closely packed glands that may be round, elongated, or have an irregular branching outline. In areas of the most abundant epithelial proliferation, the lumen is small, and the epithelium assumes almost a medullary pattern (Figure 13). The glands are rarely lined by normal tall columnar endocervical cells. Most cells are cuboidal or flattened, with granular or coarsely vacuolated cytoplasm. Occasionally, a distinct subnuclear or supranuclear vacuole is evident. The nuclei are usually round and uniform, but markedly enlarged forms with hyperchromasia and irregular contour may be seen. Incomplete squamous metaplasia is sometimes found at the surface. Mitoses are exceedingly rare and will have a normal configuration (88, 96).

The stroma between glands is sparse and edematous or congested. An inflammatory infiltrate is usually prominent and is especially rich in neutrophils, which frequently extend from the stroma through the glandular epithelium and accumulate in the lumen. Plasma cells and lymphocytes are also common and sometimes predominate. Eosinophils have been conspicuous in many patients.

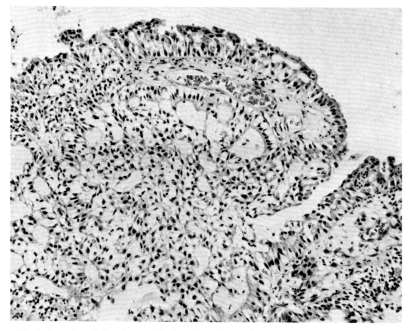

Figure 12. Microglandular hyperplasia of endocervix. Surface epithelium is stratified, with incomplete squamous metaplasia of outermost layer. Ill-defined glands are formed deeper in the mucosa.

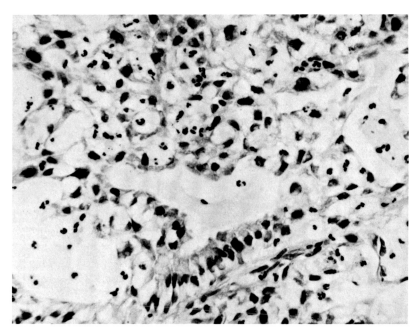

Figure 13. Margins of individual cells of microglandular hyperplasia are indistinct. Epithelial cells "melt" into periglandular stroma. Neutrophils are numerous. There is a modest variation in nuclei, with mildly atypical changes.

Taylor et al. (88) found them in large numbers in one third of their cases, and Wilkinson and Dufour found them in nearly half of their patients (92).

In comparing microglandular hyperplasia in women taking hormones with those without such a history, inflammatory infiltrate and edema tend to be more common in the hormone users (97). In addition, the extent of hyperplasia is greater in the hormone users and much more focal in the nonusers (94).

The importance of microglandular hyperplasia lies in distinguishing it from adenocarcinoma. At low power, the densely packed glands and their irregularity are worrisome. However, the uniformity of nearly all nuclei and the rarity of mitoses should restrain one from the diagnosis of cancer. Moreover, true adenocarcinoma of the endocervix, despite the existence of several patterns, does not resemble microglandular hyperplasia (98).

One especially dangerous situation is to receive a biopsy from a woman with a history of in utero stilbestrol exposure. When this history is known, one is sensitized to the possibility of clear-cell carcinoma. In one case, this diagnosis was made, but detailed study of the hysterectomy specimen led to a revision of the diagnosis to hyperplasia (92).

None of the women with microglandular hyperplasia has been reported to develop a more serious lesion during the periods of follow-up. There are now, however, several women with endocervical adenocarcinoma who have been taking oral contraceptives. One of the earliest reported cases was a well-differentiated papillary cancer with much stromal inflammation found in a woman after 4 years of hormone therapy (99). Cytologically, the neoplasm was malignant and bore no resemblance to microglandular hyperplasia. This case is of particular interest because it illustrates a paradoxic hazard of hormone therapy. The authors were deterred initially in their diagnosis of cancer because of the history of hormone usage. The patient also had squamous carcinoma in situ, and there is one other case of coexistent cervical adenocarcinoma in situ and squamous carcinoma in situ diagnosed during hormone therapy (100). It should be mentioned that concomitant adenocarcinoma in situ and squamous carcinoma in situ were reported before the availability of oral contraceptives (101).

One case of adenocarcinoma of the endocervix was detected by exfoliative cytology, revealing changes different from the mild atypia seen in the exfoliated cells of hyperplasia. The cervix included both adenocarcinoma and microglandular hyperplasia, but the authors emphasized that no cause and effect relationship should be demonstrated in their case (102). Gallup and Abell have reported five additional cases of adenocarcinoma in women less than 32 years of age, all of whom had taken oral contraceptives for 1–8 years (98). They illustrate several different patterns of adenocarcinoma but make no specific comparison of the tumors from hormone users. Dr. Murray R. Abell generously sent me the slides from these cases. Utilizing the categories of Gallup and Abell, the carcinomas included two well-differentiated adenocarcinomas of endocervical cell type and three poorly differentiated carcinomas (their medullary category). These two patterns predominated in their series regardless of whether the women were using hormones, and no histologic common denominator was recognized. Qizilbash discussed adenocarcinoma in situ of the endocervix with microinvasion. Four of his 14 cases were women taking oral contraceptives for periods of 3–10 years (103). All of these investigators are inclined to agree that oral contraceptives should not be incriminated in the pathogenesis of cervical neoplasia on the basis of the evidence thus far available.

ENDOMETRIUM

The endometrium is the uterine tissue most often altered morphologically by oral contraceptives. The changes are due mainly to the progestin, which may produce a conspicuous decidual reaction, while the glands become atrophic (glandular-stromal dissociation). The glandular epithelium passes through an initial secretory phase that peaks at Day 9 or 10 of the cycle and then becomes regressive. An occasional cell may have a slightly enlarged hyperchromatic nucleus (104), and less often an entire gland is involved. The endometrium that houses these atypical epithelial elements will contain widely scattered, predominantly atrophic glands. With this general background, the focal cytologic atypia can be placed in its proper role of having no biologic significance.

Atypical cells may be seen in the stroma, with markedly hyperchromatic and pleomorphic nuclei (Figure 14) (105–107). Atypical stromal cells may be found in endometrial aspirates and raise the question of malignancy (108). Similarly, abnormal stromal cells have been detected in exfoliated specimens (109). In most cases, the biopsy that is precipitated by these cytologic findings will disclose the general background of glandular-stromal dissociation. The atypical cells will occur in extremely small areas. As with focal epithelial alterations, when the

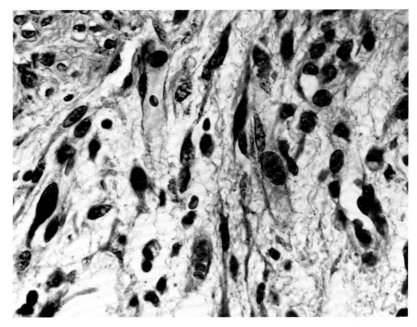

Figure 14. Pleomorphic endometrial stromal cells in patient taking combination-type oral contraceptives. Remainder of endometrium at hysterectomy showed only typical pseudodecidual alteration.

overall pattern of glandular-stromal dissociation is identified, the foci of atypical stroma can be discounted. Nonetheless, the diagnosis of endometrial stromal sarcoma has been made in a few patients, but follow-up information has not been provided (109). In other patients with atypical stromal changes in biopsy material, the abnormal cells have disappeared after hormone therapy has ceased (105).

Bona fide endometrial adenocarcinoma has been illustrated in an endometrium that exhibited stromal-glandular dissociation secondary to hormone usage (110). The concentration of neoplastic glands is in sharp contrast to the widely scattered glands of the nonneoplastic endometrium, and to their cytologic differences. In the patient with this combination, the adenocarcinoma was present prior to contraceptive steroid therapy.

The possibility that oral contraceptive hormones may be carcinogenic in the endometrium was raised by Silverberg and Makowski in 1975 (111). The details of their experience are discussed elsewhere in this volume. Several additional reports have confirmed their observation that patients taking sequential oral contraceptives are at increased risk to develop adenocarcinoma. Lyon reported four women 32–46 years of age who had been taking Oracon for periods of 4–12 years (112). One case had superficial myometrial invasion, and one had endocervical extension of cancer. Kelley et al. described three patients, 30, 37, and 48 years old, who developed well-differentiated adenocarcinoma after the use of sequential agents without interruption for 5–10 years (113). Four women taking Oracon for 8–18 years were diagnosed as cases of adenocarcinoma by Cohen and Deppe (114). One patient showed superficial myometrial invasion in the hysterectomy specimen.

The histologic appearance of the carcinomas has been unusual in two respects. Silverberg et al. found an excess of secretory and clear-cell carcinoma in hormone users when compared with young women with endometrial cancer who had never used oral contraceptives (115). It is of interest that the secretory and clear-cell components were seen in four women who had discontinued their hormone medication 8 months to 6 years prior to the diagnosis. Thus, secretory changes can be present, even in the absence of concomitant progestin administration.

The second alteration that is unusual in endometrial carcinomas is the degree of eosinophilia in the neoplastic cells. Through the courtesy of Dr. Raymond H. Kaufman, this author has been able to review nine cases of adenocarcinoma or atypical hyperplasia from patients taking Oracon for periods ranging from 4 to 8 years. Seven of these cases were described in his recent publication (116). None were infertile, and none had menstrual irregularities or evidence of Stein-Leventhal syndrome. Five of the nine cases displayed eosinophilia of at least some of the neoplastic cells, and in four of these cases, it was the predominant cell type (Figure 15). Secretory activity was abundant in one case (Figures 16 & 17).

After the relation of sequential agents to carcinoma was raised, Lyon and Frisch biopsied the endometrium of 12 asymptomatic women taking Oracon for 13–93 months (117). Seven had focal adenomatous hyperplasia, three had focal or diffuse cystic hyperplasia, and two showed a normal endometrium. The

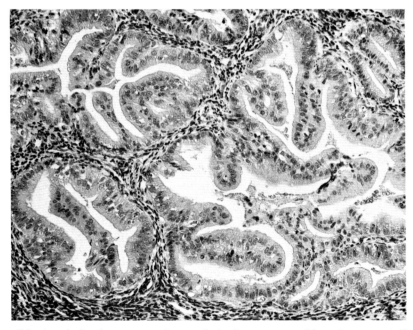

Figure 15. Atypical adenomatous hyperplasia in woman taking Oracon. Cells have abundant eosinophilic cytoplasm and papillary configuration.

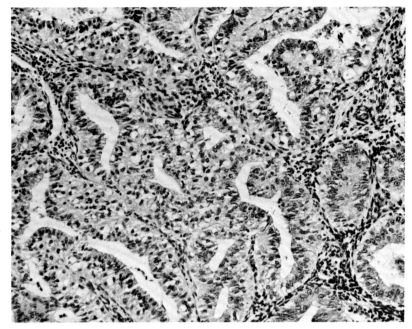

Figure 16. Well-differentiated adenocarcinoma from 44-year-old woman taking Oracon for 9 years for contraception.

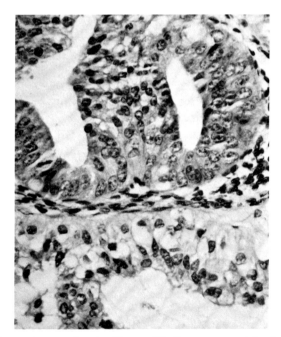

Figure 17. Same case as that in Figure 16. Secretory activity is seen in cells (*bottom*). Glands (*top*) show stratification, with moderate nuclear atypia.

129

patients were 21–32 years old, and all were nulligravida. None had a pretherapy biopsy for comparison. Nevertheless, these data would indicate that sequential agents produce hyperplastic alterations at an unexpectedly high frequency.

MYOMETRIUM

Several changes in the myometrium and in leiomyomas have been described in hormone users. The myometrium itself will enlarge and soften, especially during continuous therapy (118, 119). The cause of the enlargement is probably a combination of edema, vascular congestion, and, perhaps, muscle hypertrophy (104). Edema and congestion of the myometrium are difficult to substantiate on histologic study, but muscle hypertrophy can be seen. The myometrial fibers resemble those found in pregnancy, with abundant cytoplasm and plump light-staining nuclei (120). Although rare, these changes have been reported during cyclic therapy (121) and during long-term continuous therapy (118, 120).

Tiny myometrial nodules were described in three patients as a microscopic finding (120). The cells were uniform, with plump but bland nuclei. The cytoplasm was abundant, and the nuclei were widely separated, probably due to edema. Normal mitoses were as frequent as one per two high-power fields. Indirect evidence to suggest that these nodules may be due to the progestin component of oral contraceptives is found in the observations by Segaloff et al. (122). They treated six patients with pure progesterone and found tiny myometrial nodules in two cases. The lesions included mitotic activity, and the photographs of their myometrial nodules seem identical to the appearance in patients treated with oral contraceptives.

Oral contraceptives may produce symptomatic changes in women with preexisting myomas, but there is no evidence that the hormones induce tumor formation. Myomas can enlarge in a "startling and disturbing" manner, especially during continuous hormone therapy. Most of the growth will occur during the first 4–8 weeks and tends to stabilize after that time (123). When hormone administration ceases, the myomas shrink to pretreatment size or even smaller (118, 123, 124). Mixson and Hammond suggest that the enlargement of myomas is due to edema or vascular congestion rather than to smooth muscle proliferation (123). This contention is a reasonable hypothesis and would account for the relatively rapid return of most myomas to their original size after cessation of hormone administration.

On rare occasions, there is severe pain, necessitating surgical intervention. In this clinical setting, acute hemorrhagic necrosis of one or more myomas is found. Hemorrhagic necrosis is most often seen during continuous hormone therapy, but short-term administration can also be catastrophic. In one instance, within 5 days after the beginning of hormone administration, a myoma abruptly enlarged that had clinically been unchanged in size for at least 2 years. The accompanying severe pain was terminated by hysterectomy, and a 7-cm hemorrhagic myoma was found (125).

Hemorrhage into a myoma need not be an acutely symptomatic process, as illustrated by a 71-year-old woman receiving hormones for 1 year because of uterine bleeding. When the uterus was removed, several myomas with hemorrhagic necrosis were found, an extremely unusual event at her age (106). The pathogenesis of acute hemorrhagic necrosis is not clear. Alteration in the vascular supply of myomas is the conventional explanation, but this hypothesis has not been verified.

Myomas removed during hormone therapy may have bizarre nuclei (126, 127). We prefer the designation of "atypical myomas" for such tumors. The nuclear abnormalities range from multilobulated nuclei with a vesicular appearance to densely hyperchromatic nuclei with virtually no discernible detail (Figure 18). The latter cells may be rounded or elongated to several times the normal length of smooth muscle nuclei. The atypical nuclei are scattered focally in myomas, which elsewhere contain normal nuclei. The foci of nuclear change may involve the majority of cells in a given area or they may be individually present in a field of otherwise normal smooth muscle cells (120). The nuclear alterations have been reported in patients receiving cyclic therapy (121) or continuous therapy ranging in duration from a few months to 4 years (118, 127). The relation of the nuclear changes to hormone therapy is uncertain. Bizarre nuclei in smooth muscle tumors have been considered either as evidence of active stimulation or as a reflection of degeneration. The atypical myomas we have seen have shown no conspicuous histologic activity of either a regenerative nature (in the form of mitotic activity) or unusual degenerative foci.

The incidence of atypical myomas prior to the hormone era is difficult to assess, but some idea can be gained from one study of 1150 myomectomies (128).

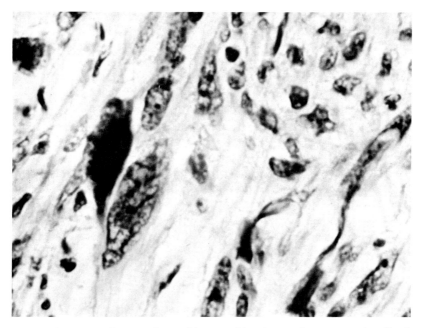

Figure 18. Leiomyoma from patient taking combination oral contraceptives for 5 years. Plump but normal-sized nuclei are seen (*upper right*). Bizarre nuclei (*left*) include dense hyperchromatic angulated nucleus and also vesicular folded nucleus with chromatin clumping.

Five of the cases were designated as leiomyosarcoma and seven as "cellular fibroid." Since all of the patients survived with myomectomy as the only therapy, it at least seems possible that these lesions were only atypical leiomyomas. Making this assumption results in an incidence of 0.96% of atypical myomas in this prehormone series. A similar line of reasoning gives a figure of 0.77% of atypical myomas in another series of 690 myomectomies performed prior to the use of oral contraceptives (129). By comparison, atypical myomas observed during oral contraceptive therapy constituted 1.2% of all myomas removed during the same span of time (120). Therefore, it must be strongly considered that the hormone therapy was merely coincidental in the patients with atypical myomas.

Whether there is a relationship of atypical myomas to hormones, it is important to separate these lesions from leiomyosarcoma. The changes in myomas in hormone-treated patients have been focal, and some might consider this lesion as "focal leiomyosarcoma within a leiomyoma" (130) or "leiomyosarcoma in situ" (131). Whichever terminology is used, when the atypical changes are confined to the myoma, the biologic behavior is that of a nonmetastasizing lesion (130–132).

Since many alterations produced by oral contraceptives mimic the changes of pregnancy, it is worth comparing the myomas of hormone users with those found during gestation. The prevalent clinical feeling that leiomyomas enlarge during pregnancy has been questioned, and the apparent enlargement may be due to an increase in the palpable surface of the tumor rather than to an increase in its mass. The various gross and microscopic changes seen in myomas removed during pregnancy include edema, hypertrophy, and numerous degenerative changes. "Pleomorphic" nuclei have been said to occur in 15% of myomas examined from pregnant uteri (133). The photographs in the relevant publication, however, fail to show the type of atypical nuclei found in bizarre leiomyomas in women taking oral contraceptives. In short, there is little resemblance between the changes in myomas of hormone users and myomas from pregnant women.

Adenomyosis can undergo typical glandular-stromal dissociation. Even with continuous therapy, however, the response is uncommonly found and is only focal (79, 119, 126).

In summary, only a small proportion of uteri removed during or after oral contraceptive therapy demonstrate morphologic changes in the myometrium or the myomas harbored therein. The temporal relationship between the initiation of hormone therapy and acute hemorrhagic necrosis of myomas seems to be satisfactory evidence of a cause and effect relationship for this rare event. The morphologic changes of bizarre myomas, however, may not be more frequent than in the prehormone era, and a definite relation to hormone usage remains to be demonstrated.

VAGINA

Vaginal adenosis has become clinically detectable during oral contraceptive therapy and has regressed when hormone usage was terminated (134). Microglandular hyperplasia occurs in vaginal adenosis, with a pattern similar to hyperplasia in the endocervix. The glands are small, closely packed and separated by little or no stroma. Incomplete squamous metaplasia may be seen (135). The problem of overinterpretation of these changes as cancer has been emphasized by Kurman and Norris (136). Robboy and Welch have noted that glycogen is present and mucin is absent in clear-cell carcinomas in the vagina, whereas the opposite is found in microglandular hyperplasia secondary to contraceptive steroids arising in vaginal adenosis (135).

BREAST

Several series and individual case reports have dealt with the pathologic findings in breast tumors from women taking oral contraceptives. Before considering these lesions, it is pertinent to review briefly some general aspects of the effect of contraceptive hormones on mammary glands.

As one would expect, very little tissue is available from normal breasts of hormone users. Autopsies of five young women who had taken oral contraceptives disclosed that three had inactive breast tissue and two had lobular hyperplasia with varying degrees of secretion (137). The parity was not given, an important oversight, because lactational changes can persist indefinitely after pregnancy (138) and would be an alternative explanation for the secretion. However, lobular hyperplasia with secretory activity indistinguishable from the normal lactating breast was found in two women taking contraceptive steroids who had never been pregnant (139). For this situation, it is reasonable to attribute the secretory effect to the hormones. One extraordinary case of lobular hyperplasia with secretion resulted in a palpable mass (140). In another study, Erb and Kallenberger biopsied the breasts of 12 women with "slight palpable alterations" and found lobular hyperplasia (adenosis) in eight of them (141). Cytologic atypia was not mentioned in any of the above reports.

Mammographic studies in women taking hormones have not revealed specific alterations (142, 143). Increased or decreased parenchymal density is perceptible in some women if mammograms are taken during hormone usage and then compared with those obtained prior to the medication (144). The differences in density may be partly a manifestation of the time at which the mammograms were taken during the menstrual cycle. An increase in the volume of the breast occurs during hormone usage that is approximately of the same degree as in spontaneous menstrual cycles in the same women (145). This difference could affect the radiographic density.

In lactating women, metabolites from a radioactive oral contraceptive were recovered in milk, but their biologic activity was not assayed (146). In one instance, metabolically active hormone was transmitted via the mother's milk to her infant son, who developed gynecomastia (147).

Galactorrhea has been reported in several patients taking oral contraceptives (148–150). The histologic changes in these breasts are not known, but since acinar formation with secretion has been seen in breast tissue from other women taking hormones, it almost certainly represents the microscopic counterpart of galactorrhea.

In turning to the tumors of the breast, fibroadenomas have been the most closely studied lesion. This is partly because fibroadenomas occur predominantly in the young adult, paralleling the years when oral contraceptives are at their peak use, and partly because early reports on five patients described a "peculiar" form of florid epithelial hyperplasia that was attributed to hormone therapy (151, 152). In other papers, however, an identical florid hyperplasia was described in a teenager (153) and in two young women who had never taken hormones (154). Most investigators have not found florid hyperplasia but only mild hyperplastic changes identical to those found in fibroadenomas from nonusers of hormones (139, 155). In one study, the frequency of bland hyperplasia was more than twice as great in fibroadenomas from users (35%) as in those from nonusers (12%) (156).

In a blind study using freshly prepared slides from age-matched controls antedating the contraceptive era, we found typical hyperplasia in 9% of fibroadenomas from users of hormones and in 7% of those in women who had never taken them (139). No qualitative difference in the hyperplasia was recognizable when the code was broken and the cases from both groups examined side by side. However, one difference was found. Acinar formation with secretion was present in four of 54 fibroadenomas from women taking hormones (Figure 19). All of these women were nulligravid, so that the lactational changes can be considered to be due to the hormones. Two other women served as their own controls, having had fibroadenomas removed before they began taking hormones and fibroadenomas excised later during the use of oral contraceptives. The stroma and epithelium were identical in the tumors removed from both patients before and during therapy (139).

Wiegenstein et al. found that 12 of 67 women with fibroadenomas had multi-

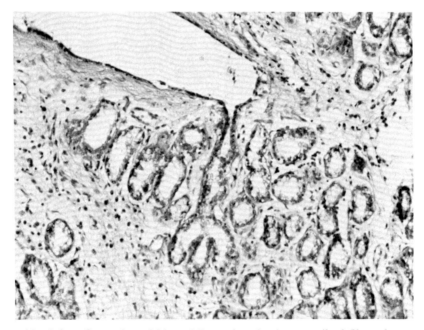

Figure 19. Acinar formation within a 1.5-cm sharply circumscribed fibroadenoma. Patient was never pregnant and was taking contraceptive hormones.

ple lesions and raised the possibility of an increase in multiple lesions in hormone users (157). This contention is not substantiated by the data of Oberman and French, who found multiple fibroadenomas in 15 of 79 women prior to the availability of hormones (158).

In addition to fibroadenomas, pure adenomas of the breast are seen almost exclusively in young women. One adenoma enlarged during the use of oral contraceptives, but neither this lesion nor five others from women who had taken hormones showed unusual histologic features when compared with several lesions from nonusers (159).

The wide spectrum of epithelial and stromal changes that characterizes fibrocystic disease makes it a more difficult lesion to evaluate than fibro-adenomas. Perhaps for this reason, no one has ascribed changes to exoge-nous hormones (153, 160–163). In one study, cases of fibrocystic disease from women taking hormones were compared with age-matched cases from nonusers. Freshly prepared slides were coded and examined without knowledge of the history. A variety of alterations, such as cysts, hyperplasia, apocrine metaplasia, adenosis, and secretory activity, were tabulated. No qualitative difference was seen. Epithelial hyperplasia was present in 32% of the breasts from nonusers and in 24% of the lesions of users of hormones (164). Similar figures (30 and 34%, respectively) were reported by Gray and Robertson (153). This frequency of hyperplasia is in accord with the categories of hyperplasia or papillomatosis of large series of fibrocystic disease reported prior to the use of oral contraception (165). No difference in the stroma was recognized between the two groups. Moreover, the age distribution of the hormone-treated patients paralleled that of a large number of women with fibrocystic disease examined prior to the hormone era.

Meyer measured the proliferative rates of epithelium in fibrocystic disease and in fibroadenomas by use of the technique of tritiated thymidine labeling. Tissue from women taking hormones had similar indices of proliferation as did tissue from nonusers (166).

Histologic observations on carcinoma of the breast from users of hormones have been reported by several authors. Gould et al. found a considerable amount of secretory activity within the carcinoma, widespread cancerization of lobules and ducts, and increased mucosubstances within the stroma around neoplastic ducts (Figures 20 & 21) (167). This combination of changes has also been noted by Norris and Taylor (168). The alterations are not specific for women taking oral contraceptives, because they may be seen in cancers from pregnant and in those from lactating women. While these changes may be characteristic of some cancers from hormone users, it must be emphasized that most carcinomas will have no distinguishing feature (169). Furthermore, diffuse cancerization of the lobules and ducts can occur in women of all ages regardless of hormone usage (170).

Penman illustrated the accumulation of large numbers of colostrum-like foam cells in the intraductal component of a cancer from a woman taking oral con-traceptives (171). No foam cells were seen in the infiltrating part of the tumor or in the metastases. Such a change is not limited to women taking hormones (172).

In addition to changes in the carcinoma itself, lobular sclerosis adjacent to carcinoma has been described in one case (173). In another study, however,

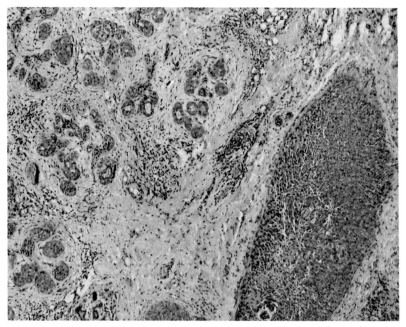

Figure 20. Carcinoma in 34-year-old woman taking oral contraceptives for 4 years. Lobules (*left*) and large ducts (*right*) are filled with cancer. Typical infiltrating ductal carcinoma was present elsewhere.

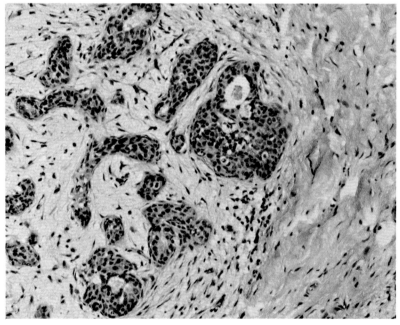

Figure 21. Higher-power photomicrograph of same case as that in Figure 20. Accumulation of secretory material is seen in some lumina. The stroma is sparsely cellular and contains abundant mucosubstance.

136

three of eight cases of cancer in young women who had never taken oral contraceptives showed some degree of lobular sclerosis (174). It is possible that young women with breast cancer who have a long history of steroid ingestion may attain a greater frequency of lobular sclerosis, but this hypothesis will require better data for its confirmation. Parenthetically, one previously reported case of breast cancer in a 28-year-old woman taking hormones for 7.5 years failed to display sclerosis (169).

Infiltrating ductal carcinoma with or without an intraductal component has been the most frequently reported form of cancer. Carcinomas of the breast should be categorized accurately, because a shift in previously reported proportions of different types of carcinoma in hormone users would be evidence of a pathogenetic influence, even if no distinctive histologic feature can be consistently identified in the individual case.

Even in the absence of consistent morphologic changes in breast cancers, the possibility exists that they may be affected by hormones. Both the estrogen and progestin components of oral contraceptives have been demonstrated in isolated cases to accelerate the growth of metastatic breast carcinoma (175). On the other hand, a premenopausal woman has exhibited a temporary response to progestin therapy (176). The use of commercially available oral contraceptive hormones in the therapy of breast cancer has been reported. Nine of 42 postmenopausal women responded, including some who had failed to respond to estrogens alone. The clinical improvement occurred in women treated at the contraceptive dose and in those who received higher doses (177).

In summary, the breast tissue of women taking contraceptive hormones does not undergo histologically distinctive changes. Nonetheless, the hormones occasionally produce lobular hyperplasia with secretory activity either in normal breast or within fibroadenomas. In addition, fibroadenomas may show a florid epithelial hyperplasia, but it is doubtful whether this appearance is qualitatively or quantitatively different from that in fibroadenomas from nonusers. Similarly, carcinomas from hormone users may show a diffuse cancerization of the ducts and lobules, but this finding is similar to the situation in cancers in other young women, especially those who are pregnant or lactating. The lack of specific alterations in women taking hormones up to the present time should not deter pathologists from continued close study of tissues from these patients. It is possible that late effects of hormone usage will eventually appear, and histologic peculiarities may still play a role in the detection of such effects.

MISCELLANEOUS

Several dozen ovaries have been obtained from women taking contraceptive steroids. The majority have shown a failure of follicular development, although the primary follicles do not seem to be altered (178). Functional ovarian cysts that require surgery are less common in women using oral contraceptives, presumably due to prevention of follicular maturation (179). There has been no report of neoplasms.

The salpinx will undergo epithelial atrophy after 18–36 months of therapy (180). Even when the epithelium is normal on light microscopic examination, scanning electron microscopy will demonstrate loss of cilia (181, 182). No atypical epithelial alteration has been reported.

One 24-year-old woman developed hyperplastic gingivitis and a pyogenic granuloma on the palate after 18 months of contraceptive hormone usage. The oral surgeon recognized this finding to be a process also seen in pregnancy and requested that she discontinue hormone usage. The gingivitis regressed, as did much of the pyogenic granuloma. The remnant of the granuloma was excised and had the usual histologic appearance of that lesion (183).

Endometriosis is often treated with combination oral contraceptives. On rare occasions, a focus of endometriosis may enlarge temporarily, as reported in one vaginal lesion that increased fourfold in size (118). In general, endometriosis reacts to oral contraceptives in a manner similar to the endometrium. The glands become atrophic and are surrounded by enlarged stromal cells that usually disappear either because of necrosis or atrophy, leaving a microscopic residue of fibrous tissue and histiocytes. Endometriomas of the ovary as large as 12 cm in diameter have regressed during hormone therapy (184). Importantly, endometriomas do not seem to enlarge or rupture during therapy. Occasionally, the decidual reaction will persist and form a thick lining to the cyst (Figure 22).

SUMMARY

A concern for the possible carcinogenic effects of oral contraceptive hormones has been expressed repeatedly since their introduction in 1960. This concern is founded in great part on data obtained in experimental animals, which have

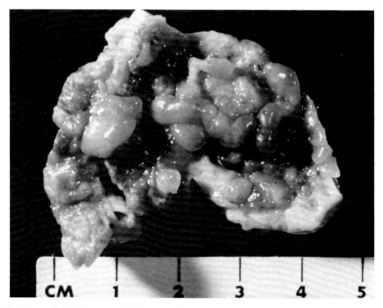

Figure 22. Part of the inner wall of an endometrial cyst of the ovary. Patient had been on combination contraceptive therapy continuously for 7 months for endometriosis. Lobulated portion of cyst lining is due to pseudodecidual reaction.

linked estrogens to the induction and/or enhanced growth of tumors in the breast and female genital organs. In humans, however, the number of tumors possibly related to oral contraceptives has proven to be few (thus far) in view of the millions of women who have used these agents. Ironically, the largest group of tumors that appear to be associated with hormones has not been in the breast or genital tract but rather in the liver.

REFERENCES

1. Fechner RE: Benign hepatic lesions and orally administered contraceptives. A report of seven cases and a critical analysis of the literature. Human Pathol 8:255, 1977.

2. Baum JK, Holtz F, Bookstein JJ, et al: Possible association between benign hepatomas and oral contraceptives. Lancet 2:926, 1973.

3. Horvath E, Kovacs K, Ross RC: Ultrastructural findings in a well-differentiated hepatoma. Digestion 7:74, 1972.

4. Chan CK, Detmer DE: Proper management of hepatic adenoma associated with oral contraceptives. Surg Gynecol Obstet 144:703, 1977.

5. Keifer WS Jr, Scott JC: Liver neoplasms and the oral contraceptives. Amer J Obstet Gynecol 128:448, 1977.

6. Stauffer JQ, Lapinski MW, Honold DJ, et al: Focal nodular hyperplasia of the liver and intrahepatic hemorrhage in young women on oral contraceptives. Ann Intern Med 83:301, 1975.

7. Tountas C, Paraskevas G, Deligeorgi H: Benign hepatoma and oral contraceptives. Lancet 1:1351, 1974.

8. Berg JW, Ketelaar RJ, Rose EF, et al: Hepatomas and oral contraceptives. Lancet 2:349, 1974.

9. Ishak KG, Rabin L: Benign tumors of the liver. Med Clin N Amer 59:995, 1975.

10. Edmondson HA, Henderson B, Benton B: Liver-cell adenomas associated with use of oral contraceptives. N Engl J Med 294:470, 1976.

11. Model DG, Fox JA, Jones RW: Multiple hepatic adenomas associated with an oral contraceptive. Lancet 1:865, 1975.

12. Hilliard JL, Graham DY, Spjut HJ: Hepatic adenoma: a possible complication of oral contraceptive therapy. South Med J 69:683, 1976.

13. Contostavlos DL: Benign hepatomas and oral contraceptives. Lancet 2:1200, 1973.

14. Antoniades K, Campbell WN, Hecksher RH, et al: Liver cell adenomas and oral contraceptives. Double tumor development. J Amer Med Ass 234:628, 1975.

15. Antoniades K, Brooks CE Jr: Hemoperitoneum from liver cell adenoma in a patient on oral contraceptives. Surgery 77:137, 1975.

16. Galloway SJ, Casarella WJ, Lattes R, et al: Minimal deviation hepatoma. Amer J Roentgenol Radium Ther Nucl Med 125:184, 1975.

17. Nissen ED, Kent DR: Liver tumors and oral contraceptives. Obstet Gynecol 46:460, 1975.

18. Mays ET, Christopherson WM, Barrows GH: Focal nodular hyperplasia of the liver. Possible relationship to oral contraceptives. Amer J Clin Pathol 61:735, 1974.

19. O'Sullivan JP, Wilding RP: Liver hamartomas in patients on oral contraceptives. Brit Med J 2:7, 1974.

20. Christopherson WM, Mays ET, Barrows G: A clinicopathologic study of steroid-related liver tumors. Amer J Surg Pathol 1:31, 1977.

21. Center for Disease Control. Morbid Mortal Weekly Rep 26:293, 1977.

22. Kay S, Schatzki PF: Ultrastructure of a benign liver cell adenoma. Cancer 28:755, 1971.

23. Kay S: Personal communication, 1975.

24. Davis JB, Schenken JR, Zimmerman O: Massive hemoperitoneum from rupture of benign hepatocellular adenoma. Surgery **73**:181, 1973.

25. Schenken JR: Hepatocellular adenoma: relationship to oral contraceptives? J Amer Med Ass **236**:559, 1976.

26. Albritton DR, Tompkins RK, Longmire WP: Hepatic cell adenomas: a report of four cases. Ann Surg **180**:14, 1974.

27. Albritton DR: Personal communication, 1975.

28. Motsay GJ, Gamble WG: Clinical experience with hepatic adenomas. Surg Gynecol Obstet **134**:415, 1972.

29. Gamble WG: Personal communication, 1975.

30. Ameriks JA, Thompson NW, Frey CF, et al: Hepatic cell adenomas, spontaneous liver rupture, and oral contraceptives. Arch Surg **110**:548, 1975.

31. Goldstein HM, Neiman HL, Mena E, et al: Angiographic findings in benign liver cell tumors. Radiology **110**:339, 1974.

32. McAvoy JM, Tompkins RK, Longmire WP: Benign hepatic tumors and their association with oral contraceptives. Case reports and survey of the literature. Arch Surg **111**:761, 1976.

33. Nissen ED, Kent DR, Nissen SE: Etiologic factors in the pathogenesis of liver tumors associated with oral contraceptives. Amer J Obstet Gynecol **127**:61, 1977.

34. Edmondson HA: Tumors of the liver and intrahepatic bile ducts, *Atlas of Tumor Pathology,* Washington, DC, Armed Forces Institute of Pathology, 1958, section VII, fascicle 25.

35. Ackerman LV, Rosai J: Surgical Pathology. St. Louis, CV Mosby, 1974, p. 533, 5th edit.

36. Knowles DM, Wolff M, Casarella WJ: Hepatic cell adenomas. Arch Surg **110**:1154, 1975.

37. Knowles DM II, Kaye GI, Goodman GC: Nodular regenerative hyperplasia of the liver. Gastroenterology **69**:746, 1975.

38. Sorensen TIA, Baden H: Benign hepatocellular tumors. Scand J Gastroenterol **10**:113, 1975.

39. Begg CF, Berry WH: Isolated nodules of regenerative hyperplasia of the liver. Amer J Clin Pathol **23**:447, 1953.

40. Kwittken J: Hamartoma of the liver. NY State J Med **67**:3254, 1967.

41. Christopherson WM, Mays ET: Liver tumors and contraceptive steroids: experience with the first one hundred registry patients. J Nat Cancer Inst **58**:167, 1977.

42. Catalano PW, Early ME, Topolosky HW, et al: Focal nodular hyperplasia of the liver: report of six patients. Concepts of surgical management. Cancer **39**:587, 1977.

43. Benz EJ, Baggenstoss AH: Focal cirrhosis of the liver: its relation to the so-called hamartoma (adenoma, benign hepatoma). Cancer **6**:743, 1953.

44. Alpert LI: Veno-occlusive disease of the liver associated with oral contraceptives: case report and review of literature. Human Pathol **7**:709, 1976.

45. Mays ET, Christopherson WM, Mahr MM, et al: Hepatic changes in young women ingesting contraceptive steroids. Hepatic hemorrhage and primary hepatic tumors. J Amer Med Ass **235**:730, 1976.

46. Winkler K, Poulsen H: Liver disease with periportal sinusoidal dilatation: a possible complication of contraceptive steroids. Scand J Gastroenterol **10**:699, 1975.

47. Frederick WC, Howard RG, Spatola S: Spontaneous rupture of the liver in patient using contraceptive pills. Arch Surg **108**:93, 1974.

48. Edmondson HA, Reynolds TB, Henderson B, et al: Regression of liver cell adenomas associated with oral contraceptives. Ann Intern Med **86**:180, 1977.

49. Fechner RE, Roehm JOF Jr: Angiographic and pathologic correlations of hepatic focal nodular hyperplasia. Amer J Surg Pathol **1**:217, 1977.

50. Lansing PB, McQuitty JT, Bradburn DM: Benign liver tumors. What is their relationship to oral contraceptives? Amer Surg **42**:744, 1976.

51. Kalra TMS, Mangla JC, DePapp EW: Benign hepatic tumors and oral contraceptive pills. Amer J Med **61**:871, 1976.

52. Baek S, Sloane CE, Futterman SC: Benign liver cell adenoma associated with use of oral contraceptive agents. Ann Surg **183**:239, 1976.

53. Ross D, Pina J, Mirza M, et al: Regression of focal nodular hyperplasia after discontinuation of oral contraceptives. Ann Intern Med **85**:203, 1976.

54. Andersen PH, Packer JT: Hepatic adenoma. Observations after estrogen withdrawal. Arch Surg **111**:898, 1976.

55. Brander WL, Vosnides G, Ogg CS, et al: Multiple hepatocellular tumours in a patient treated with oral contraceptives. Virch Arch A Pathol Anat Histol **370**:69, 1976.

56. Gonzales-Angulo A, Aznar-Ramos R, Marquez-Monter H, et al: The ultrastructure of liver cells in women under steroid therapy. I. Normal pregnancy and trophoblastic growths. Acta Endocrinol **65**:193, 1970.

57. Phillips MJ, Langer B, Stone R, et al: Benign liver cell tumors. Classification and ultrastructural pathology. Cancer **32**:463, 1973.

58. Rogers LA, Morris HP, Fouts JR: The effect of phenobarbital on drug metabolic enzyme activity, ultrastructure, and growth of a "minimal deviation" hepatoma (Morris 7800). J Pharmacol Exp Ther **157**:227, 1967.

59. Bhagwat AG, Ross RC: Hepatic intramitochondrial crystalloids. Arch Pathol **91**:70, 1971.

60. Perez V, Gorosdisch S, Demartire J, et al: Oral contraceptives: long-term use produces fine structural changes in liver mitochondria. Science **165**:805, 1969.

61. Martinez-Manautou J, Aznar-Ramos R, Bautista-O'Farrill J, et al: The ultrastructure of liver cells in women under steroid therapy. II. Contraceptive therapy. Acta Endocrinol **65**:207, 1970.

62. Bhagwat AG, Ross RC, Currie DJ: Ultrastructure of normal human liver. Arch Pathol **93**:227, 1972.

63. Lynn JA: Hepatic ultrastructural variations in apparently "normal" humans (Abst.). Lab Invest **20**:594, 1969.

64. Roth GJ, Trump BF, Smuckler EA: Occurrence and nature of mitochondrial matrix striations (Abst.). J Cell Biol **23**:79A, 1964.

65. Wills EJ: Crystalline structures in the mitochondria of normal human liver parenchymal cells. J Cell Biol **24**:511, 1965.

66. Hermann RE, David TE: Spontaneous rupture of the liver caused by hepatomas. Surgery **74**:715, 1973.

67. Hermann RE: Personal communication, 1976.

68. Davis M, Portmann B, Searle M, et al: Histological evidence of carcinoma in a hepatic tumor associated with oral contraceptives. Brit Med J **4**:496, 1975.

69. O'Sullivan JP, Rosswick RP: Oral contraceptives and malignant hepatic tumours. Lancet **1**:1124, 1976.

70. Knowles DM II, Wolff M: Focal nodular hyperplasia of the liver. A clinical pathologic study and review of the literature. Human Pathol **7**:533, 1976.

71. Shojania NG, Hogg GR: Isolated liver nodules. Gastroenterology **69**:28, 1975.

72. Meyer P, Livolsi VA, Cornog JL: Hepatoblastoma associated with an oral contraceptive. Lancet **2**:1387, 1974.

73. Carter R: Hepatoblastoma in the adult. Cancer **23**:191, 1969.

74. El-Domeiri AA, Huvos AG, Goldsmith HS, et al: Primary malignant tumors of the liver. Cancer **27**:7, 1971.

75. Vessey MP, Kay CR, Baldwin JA, et al: Oral contraceptives and benign liver tumours. Brit Med J **1**:1064, 1977.

76. Grabowski M, Stenram U, Bergqvist A: Focal nodular hyperplasia of the liver, benign hepatomas, oral contraceptives and other drugs affecting the liver. Acta Pathol Microbiol Scand **83A**:615, 1975.

77. Whitehead N, Reyner F, Lindenbaum J: Megaloblastic changes in the cervical epithelium: association with oral contraceptive therapy and reversal with folic acid. J Amer Med Ass **226**:1421, 1973.

78. Ayre JE, Hillemanns HG, LeGuerrier JM, et al: Influence of norethynodrel and mestranol upon cervical dysplasia and carcinoma in situ. Obstet Gynecol **28**:90, 1966.

79. Dito WR, Batsakis JG: Norethynodrel-treated endometriosis: a morphologic and histochemical study. Obstet Gynecol **18**:1, 1961.

80. Maqueo M, Azuela JC, Calderon JJ, et al: Morphology of the cervix in women treated with synthetic progestins. Amer J Obstet Gynecol **96**:994, 1966.

81. Carbia E, Rubio-Linares G, Alvarado-Duran A, et al: Histologic study of the uterine cervix during oral contraception with ethynodiol diacetate and mestranol. Obstet Gynecol **35**:381, 1970.

82. Zanartu J: Effect of synthetic oral gestagens on cervical mucus and sperm penetration. Int J Fertil **9**:225, 1964.

83. Roland M, Smith JJ, Romney SL: New synthetic progestational compound in infertility. Int J Fertil **5**:8, 1960.

84. Moghissi KS: Cyclic change in cervical mucus in normal and progestin-treated women. Fertil Steril **17**:663, 1966.

85. Kellet WW III, Hester LL Jr, Spicer SS, et al: Effects of a sequential oral contraceptive on endocervical carbohydrate histochemistry. Obstet Gynecol **34**:536, 1969.

86. Cohen MR, Perez-Pelaez M: The effect of norethindrone acetate, ethinyl estradiol, clomiphene citrate, and dydrogesterone on spinnbarkeit. Fertil Steril **16**:141, 1965.

87. Cohen MR: Cervical mucorrhea and spinnbarkeit in patients taking norethindrone plus mestranol (Norinyl 1 mgm). Fertil Steril **19**:405, 1968.

88. Taylor HB, Irey NS, Norris HJ: Atypical endocervical hyperplasia in women taking oral contraceptives. J Amer Med Ass **202**:637, 1967.

89. Graham J, Graham R, Hirabayashi K: Reversible "cancer" and the contraceptive pill. Report of a case. Obstet Gynecol **31**:190, 1968.

90. Candy J, Abell MR: Progestogen-induced adenomatous hyperplasia of the uterine cervix. J Amer Med Ass **203**:323, 1968.

91. Fechner RE: The surgical pathology of the reproductive system and breast during oral contraceptive therapy. Pathol Annu **6**:103, 1971.

92. Wilkinson E, Dufour DR: Pathogenesis of microglandular hyperplasia of the cervix uteri. Obstet Gynecol **47**:189, 1976.

93. Mingeot R, Fievez C: Endocervical changes with the use of synthetic steroids. Obstet Gynecol **44**:53, 1974.

94. Nichols TM, Fidler HK: Microglandular hyperplasia in cervical cone biopsies taken for suspicious and positive cytology. Amer J Clin Pathol **56**:424, 1971.

95. Kline TS, Holland M, Wemple D: Atypical cytology with contraceptive hormone medication. Amer J Clin Pathol **53**:215, 1970.

96. Kyriakos M, Kempson RL, Konikov NF: A clinical and pathologic study of endocervical lesions associated with oral contraceptives. Cancer **22**:99, 1968.

97. Govan ADT, Black WP, Sharp JL: Aberrant glandular polypi of the uterine cervix associated with contraceptive pills: pathology and pathogenesis. J Clin Pathol **22**:84, 1969.

98. Gallup DG, Abell MR: Invasive adenocarcinoma of the uterine cervix. Obstet Gynecol **49**:596, 1977.

99. Talbert JR, Sherry JB: Adenocarcinoma-like lesion of cervix—a "pill-induced" problem? Amer J Obstet Gynecol **105**:117, 1969.

100. Lauchlan SC, Penner DW: Simultaneous adenocarcinoma in situ and epidermoid carcinoma in situ. Cancer **20**:2250, 1967.

101. Friedell GH, McKay DG: Adenocarcinoma in situ of the endocervix. Cancer **6**:887, 1953.

102. Czernobilsky B, Kessler I, Lancet M: Cervical adenocarcinoma in a woman on long-term contraceptives. Obstet Gynecol **43**:517, 1974.

103. Qizilbash AH: In situ and microinvasive adenocarcinoma of the uterine cervix. Amer J Clin Pathol **64**:155, 1975.

104. Azzopardi JG, Zayid I: Synthetic progestogen-oestrogen therapy and uterine changes. J Clin Pathol **20**:731, 1967.

105. Cruz-Aquino M, Shenker L, Blaustein A: Pseudosarcoma of the endometrium. Obstet Gynecol **29**:93, 1967.

106. Dockerty MB, Smith RA, Symmonds RE: Pseudomalignant endometrial changes induced by administration of new synthetic progestins. Mayo Clin Proc **34**:321, 1959.

107. Ober WB: Effects of oral and intrauterine administration of contraceptives on the uterus. Human Pathol **8**:513, 1977.

108. Ishizuka Y, Shigenaga Y: Cytologic effects of progestogens on the endometrium of normally menstruating women. Acta Cytol **12**:146, 1968.

109. Song J, Mark MS, Lawler MP Jr: Endometrial changes in women receiving oral contraceptives. Amer J Obstet Gynecol **107**:717, 1970.

110. Fechner RE, Kaufman RH: Endometrial adenocarcinoma in Stein-Leventhal syndrome. Cancer **34**:444, 1974.

111. Silverberg SG, Makowski EL: Endometrial carcinoma in young women taking oral contraceptive agents. Obstet Gynecol **46**:503, 1975.

112. Lyon FA: The development of adenocarcinoma of the endometrium in young women receiving long term sequential oral contraception. Amer J Obstet Gynecol **46**:503, 1975.

113. Kelley HW, Miles PA, Buster JE, et al: Adenocarcinoma of the endometrium in women taking sequential oral contraceptives. Obstet Gynecol **47**:200, 1976.

114. Cohen CJ, Deppe G: Endometrial carcinoma and oral contraceptive agents. Obstet Gynecol **49**:390, 1977.

115. Silverberg SG, Makowski EL, Roche WD: Endometrial carcinoma in women under 40 years of age: Comparison of cases in oral contraceptive users and non-users. Cancer **39**:592, 1977.

116. Kaufman RH, Reeves KO, Dougherty CM: Severe atypical endometrial changes and sequential contraceptive use. J Amer Med Ass **236**:923, 1976.

117. Lyon FA, Frisch MJ: Endometrial abnormalities occurring in young women on long term sequential oral contraception. Obstet Gynecol **47**:639, 1976.

118. Andrews MC, Andrews WC, Strauss AF: Effects of progestin-induced pseudopregnancy on endometriosis: clinical and microscopic studies. Amer J Obstet Gynecol **78**:776, 1959.

119. Riva HL, Kawasaki DM, Messinger AJ: Further experience with norethynodrel in treatment of endometriosis. Obstet Gynecol **19**:111, 1962.

120. Fechner RE: Atypical leiomyomas and synthetic progestin therapy. Amer J Clin Pathol **49**:697, 1968.

121. Ryan GM Jr, Craig J, Reid DE: Histology of the uterus and ovaries after long-term cyclic norethynodrel therapy. Amer J Obstet Gynecol **90**:715, 1964.

122. Segaloff A, Weed JC, Sternberg WH, et al: The progesterone therapy of human uterine leiomyomas. J Clin Endocrinol **9**:1273, 1949.

123. Mixson WT, Hammond DO: Response of fibromyomas to a progestin. Amer J Obstet Gynecol **82**:754, 1961.

124. Lebherz TB, Fobes CD: Management of endometriosis with norprogesterone. Amer J Obstet Gynecol **81**:102, 1961.

125. Briscoe CC: Acute hemorrhagic degeneration of a leiomyoma following norethindrone acetate. Report of a case. Obstet Gynecol **23**:279, 1964.

126. Goldzieher JW, Maqueo M, Ricaud L, et al: Induction of degenerative changes of uterine myomas by high-dosage progestin therapy. Amer J Obstet Gynecol **96**:1078, 1966.

127. Prakash S, Scully RE: Sarcoma-like pseudopregnancy changes in uterine leiomyomas. Report of a case resulting from prolonged norethindrone therapy. Obstet Gynecol **24**:106, 1964.

128. Davids AM: Myomectomy: surgical technique and results in a series of 1,150 cases. Amer J Obstet Gynecol **63**:592, 1952.

129. Langstadt JR, Javert CT: Sarcoma and myomectomy. Cancer **8**:1142, 1955.

130. Silverberg SG: Leiomyosarcoma of the uterus. A clinicopathologic study. Obstet Gynecol **38**:613, 1971.

131. Przybora LA: Leiomyosarcoma in situ of the uterus. Cancer **14**:483, 1961.

132. Christopherson WM, Williamson EO, Gray LA: Leiomyosarcoma of the uterus. Cancer **29:**1512, 1972.

133. Hertig AT, Gore H: Tumors of the female sex organs. Part 2, Tumors of the Vulva, Vagina and Uterus. Washington DC, Armed Forces Institute of Pathology, 1960, p. 235, section IX, fascicle 33.

134. Strand CL, Windhager HA, Kim EH: Prompt regression of cystic vaginal adenosis following cessation of oral contraceptive therapy. Amer J Clin Pathol **64:**483, 1975.

135. Robboy SJ, Welch WR: Microglandular hyperplasia in vaginal adenosis associated with oral contraceptives and prenatal diethylstilbestrol exposure. Obstet Gynecol **49:**430, 1977.

136. Kurman RJ, Norris HJ: Adenosis. Obstet Gynecol **46:**373, 1975.

137. Irey NS, Manion WC, Taylor HB: Vascular lesions in women taking oral contraceptives. Arch Pathol **89:**1, 1970.

138. Frantz VK, Pickren JW, Melcher GW, et al: Incidence of chronic cystic disease in so-called "normal breasts." A study based on 225 postmortem examinations. Cancer **4:**762, 1951.

139. Fechner RE: Fibroadenomas in patients receiving oral contraceptives: a clinical and pathologic study. Amer J Clin Pathol **53:**857, 1970.

140. Dito WR, Batsakis JG: Norethynodrel-treated endometriosis: a morphologic and histochemical study. Obstet Gynecol **18:**1, 1961.

141. Erb H, Kallenberger A: The action of an oral high-dosed oestrogen-progestagen combination on the human breast. Acta Endocrinol **70:**143, 1972.

142. Bilbao MK: Mammography in normal women: "blind" study of Enovid effects. Amer J Roentgenol Radium Ther Nucl Med **102:**933, 1968.

143. McBride WG, MacMillian IS, Heber KR: A comparative study of adverse effects of oral contraceptives. Med J Aust **2:**246, 1974.

144. Brezina K, Janisch H, Muller-Tyl E: Das Mammogramm unter Kontrazeptiva. Wien Klin Wochschr **85:**785, 1973.

145. Milligan D, Drife JO, Short RV: Changes in breast volume during normal menstrual cycle and after oral contraceptives. Brit Med J **4:**494, 1975.

146. Laumas KR, Malkani PK, Bhatnagar S, et al: Radioactivity in the breast milk of lactating women after oral administration of ^{3}H-norethynodrel. Amer J Obstet Gynecol **98:**411, 1967.

147. Curtis EM: Oral contraceptive feminization of normal male infant. Obstet Gynecol **23:**295, 1964.

148. Gregg WI: Galactorrhea after contraceptive hormones. N Engl J Med **274:**1432, 1966.

149. Rosen SW, Gahres EE: Nonpuerperal galactorrhea and the contraceptive pill. Obstet Gynecol **29:**730, 1967.

150. Schachner SH: Galactorrhea subsequent to contraceptive hormones. N Engl J Med **275:**1138, 1966.

151. Brown JM: Histological modification of fibroadenoma of the breast associated with oral hormonal contraceptives. Med J Aust **1:**276, 1970.

152. Goldenberg VE, Wiegenstein L, Mottet NK: Florid breast fibroadenomas in patients taking hormonal oral contraceptives. Amer J Clin Pathol **49:**52, 1968.

153. Gray LA, Robertson RW: Estrogens, the pill, and the breast, in *Early Breast Cancer. Detection and Treatment*, Gallager HS (ed.), New York, John Wiley & Sons, 1975, p. 27.

154. Vessey MP, Doll R, Sutton PM: Oral contraceptives and breast neoplasia: a retrospective study. Brit Med J **3:**719, 1972.

155. Prechtel K, Seidel H: Brustdrüsenveränderungen nach Langzeitbehandlung mit sogenannten Ovulationshemmern. Verh Dtsch Ges Pathol **56:**529, 1972.

156. Prechtel K, Seidel H: Der Einfluss oraler Steroidkontrazeptiva auf das Fibroadenom der Mamma. Dtsch Med Wochschr **98:**698, 1973.

157. Wiegenstein L, Tank R, Gould VE: Multiple breast fibroadenomas in women on hormonal contraceptives. N Engl J Med **284:**676, 1971.

158. Oberman HA, French AJ: Chronic fibrocystic disease of the breast. Surg Gynecol Obstet **112:**647, 1961.

159. Hertel BF, Zaloudek C, Kempson RL: Breast adenomas. Cancer **37:**2891, 1976.

160. Ariel IM: Enovid therapy (norethynodrel with mestranol) for fibrocystic disease. Amer J Obstet Gynecol **117:**453, 1973.

161. Prechtel K: Ovulationshemmer und Brustdrüsenveränderungen bei Frauen im geschlechtsreifen Alter. Munch Med Wochschr **111:**2443, 1969.

162. Vessey MP, Doll R, Sutton PM: Investigation of the possible relationship between oral contraceptives and benign and malignant breast disease. Cancer **28:**1395, 1971.

163. Zanartu J, Onetto E, Medina E, et al: Mammary gland nodules in women under continuous exposure to progestagens. Contraception **7:**203, 1973.

164. Fechner RE: Fibrocystic disease in women receiving oral contraceptive hormones. Cancer **25:**1332, 1970.

165. McLaughlin CW Jr, Schenken JR, Tamisiea JX: A study of precancerous hyperplasia and noninvasive papillary carcinoma of the breast. Ann Surg **153:**735, 1961.

166. Meyer JS: Cell proliferation in normal human breast ducts, fibroadenomas, and other ductal hyperplasias measured by nuclear labeling with tritiated thymidine. Effects of menstrual phase, age, and oral contraceptive hormones. Human Pathol **8:**67, 1977.

167. Gould VE, Wolff M, Mottet NK: Morphologic features of mammary carcinomas in women taking hormonal contraceptives. Amer J Clin Pathol **57:**139, 1972.

168. Norris HJ, Taylor HB: Carcinoma of the breast in women less than thirty years old. Cancer **26:**953, 1970.

169. Fechner RE: Breast cancer during oral contraceptive therapy. Cancer **26:**1204, 1970.

170. Fechner RE: Ductal carcinoma involving the lobule of the breast. A source of confusion with lobular carcinoma in situ. Cancer **28:**274, 1971.

171. Penman HG: The effect of oral contraceptives on the histology of carcinoma of the breast. J Pathol **101:**66, 1970.

172. Taylor HB: Oral contraceptives and pathologic changes in the breast. Cancer **28:**1388, 1971.

173. Kovi J, Viola MV: Oral contraceptives and breast histology. J Amer Med Ass **223:**802, 1973.

174. Fechner RE: Oral contraceptive effects on the breast. J Amer Med Ass **224:**249, 1973.

175. Emerson K Jr, Jessiman AG: Hormonal influences on the growth and progression of cancer. Test for hormone dependency in mammary and prostatic cancer. N Engl J Med **254:**252, 1956.

176. Stoll BA: Hormonal Management in Breast Cancer, Philadelphia, JB Lippincott, 1969, p. 73.

177. Stoll BA: Effect of Lyndiol, an oral contraceptive, on breast cancer. Brit Med J **1:**150, 1967.

178. Maqueo M, Rice-Wray E, Calderon JJ, et al: Ovarian morphology after prolonged use of steroid contraceptive agents. Contraception **5:**177, 1972.

179. Ory H: Functional ovarian cysts and oral contraceptives: negative association confirmed surgically. J Amer Med Ass **228:**68, 1974.

180. Mahgoub SE, Karim M, Ammar R: Long-term effects of injected progestogens on the morphology of human oviducts. J Reprod Med **8:**288, 1972.

181. Fredricsson B, Bjorkman N: Morphologic alterations in the human oviduct epithelium induced by contraceptive steroids. Fertil Steril **24:**19, 1973.

182. Patek E, Nilsson L, Johannisson E, et al: Scanning electron microscopic study of the human fallopian tube, Report III: The effect of mid pregnancy and of various steroids. Fertil Steril **24:**31, 1973.

183. Kaufman AY: An oral contraceptive as an etiologic factor in producing hyperplastic gingivitis and a neoplasm of the pregnancy tumor type. Oral Surg Oral Med Oral Pathol **28:**666, 1969.

184. Gunning JE, Moyer D: The effect of medroxy-progesterone acetate on endometriosis in the human female. Fertil Steril **18:**759, 1967.

Panel Discussion: Contraception and Cancer

Question: Dr. Stadel, in your review of the literature, was there any information concerning the incidence of breast carcinoma in women on oral contraceptives whose mothers had been diagnosed as having breast carcinoma?

Dr. Stadel: I think that is one of the most important issues that needs to be studied but has not been presented explicitly. The only prospective data that are available are from the two large British cohort studies: the Royal College of General Practitioners study headed by Dr. Kay in Manchester and the community study conducted by Dr. Vessey in Oxford. Neither of these studies has sufficient cases to begin to estimate risks by any degree of accuracy. I believe Martin Vessey's cohort study has three cases of breast cancer thus far, so it is not possible at the present time to evaluate this relationship. In fact, I think it is more likely that the earliest answer regarding this relationship will come from further case control studies, examining interactions between reported oral contraceptive use and family history as a complex of factors, where one would look for an effect of oral contraceptives in the stratum of both cases and controls who had a family history. I think it will be a very long time before we get data from prospective studies to address this issue.

Question: What is unique about Oracon that it would cause the problems it appeared to produce? Does it have a unique hormonal principle or is it produced in a unique way such that it would have a toxic effect on the endometrium?

Dr. Silverberg: We are not really aware that there was anything particularly unique about it. The estrogen in Oracon is ethynylestradiol, but that compound is not unique to Oracon nor has ethynylestradiol in any other compound been shown to be associated with any type of cancer. It is, however, a relatively strong estrogen combined with a relatively weak progestogen. I think that Oracon comprised about 60–65% of the sequential market. Since it was the most popular sequential, one would indeed expect it to be the drug that was most frequently implicated among the sequentials in association with any side effect. Certainly, 60–65% was not the overwhelming 90–95% that we saw. Nevertheless, we were dealing with very small numbers of cases, and I'm not even sure that the overwhelming preponderance of Oracon was indeed significant. I just mention it because, on the other hand, we found very little to implicate any of the other sequential oral contraceptives.

Question: Dr. Silverberg, did you have any time or duration of use statistics regarding predilection for this drug?

Dr. Silverberg: Because we didn't have any population-based denominator, it wouldn't really have meant anything. The duration of contraceptive usage by patients in the Registry went from 6 months to 10 years. All of the ones that were under a year had been placed in the separate category that we threw out in considering the pills as possible etiologic agents. In terms of the others, I don't think there was any well-defined pattern distinguishing the patients on sequentials from those on combined agents. As I mentioned, older women tended to have been taking the pills longer.

Dr. Morris: Several years ago, Ed Makowski asked me if we had any carcinomas of the endometrium in patients under 40 who had been on sequentials. I didn't answer the letter because we didn't have any. Then this article was published, and I was astounded because we have seen more than 350 patients under the age of 40 in Connecticut who have not been on oral sequential contraceptives. Could the fact that the Connecticut River has fumes be responsible for this much higher incidence? How can you establish an etiologic relationship unless you have a control group?

Dr. Silverberg: You had 350 cases of endometrial carcinoma under the age of 40?

Dr. Morris: I think there were 369 in the state.

Dr. Silverberg: And how many cases do you have overall, because you should be able to multiply that by 40. If you look in the literature, only about 2.5% of cases of endometrial cancer occur in women under age 40. Does that work out?

Dr. Morris: Somewhere between 5000 and 7000.

Dr. Silverberg: One of the points that I have been emphasizing is that we don't know the denominator. If expressed in its broadest terms, the denominator is comprised of the approximately 17 million women who are taking or have taken oral contraceptive agents. Certainly, 30 cases of endometrial carcinoma is a very small drop in the bucket, and we have no way of knowing how many more cases were not reported to us. Obviously, when you are dealing with Registry material—the same is true of the liver tumor Registry or any other Registry that just advertises for cases—you are subject to the whims of people who decide to submit or not to submit their cases to you. We did have two well-defined groups, the patients who were taking sequentials and the patients who were taking combined agents, so at least we could compare those two groups. We thought that the differences were very suggestive, but we certainly could not make a statement—nor have we ever made a statement—that sequential oral contraceptives cause cancer, because our data are insufficient to justify that conclusion.

Dr. Morris: We have the same problem with the liver tumors reported because the patient was on oral contraceptives. I looked up the liver tumors prior to the advent of oral contraceptives. They are mostly in women and were blamed on tight corsets if you go back to the turn of the century.

Dr. Silverberg: Dr. Bloustein, do you have any comment on that?

Dr. Bloustein: Obviously, tight corsets are not to be blamed.

Dr. Silverberg: Dr. Bloustein doesn't like tight corsets.

Dr. Stadel: In a recent study from the Center for Disease Control, Dr. Howard Ory reported to the Society of Epidemiologic Research a couple of months back that in liver cell adenomas, for more than 7 years of oral contraceptive use, the relative risk was 500. Given that this was a study in which cases were matched to controls on a population basis, there have been very few situations of a case control study where the evidence for etiology is as strong as it is in this case.

Dr. Morris: I am only questioning the methodology, because you do not have a comparative group unless you take all of the cases under age 40 in the United States and then relate that number to the total number of women who are taking this particular contraceptive combination.

Dr. Stadel: My organization is currently soliciting a case control study of breast, endometrial, and ovarian cancer in women of reproductive age. One of our hopes is to have more control data concerning the various risk factors in endometrial cancer in young women.

Dr. Major: We have seen three endometrial carcinomas in the last four years in women under age 40, one of which was a stage II lesion that was treated effectively with extensive radical therapy; the other two, which were stage I, had very poorly differentiated lesions, and both patients are dead. They showed early evidence of systemic disease. None of these three had any history of oral contraceptives. Thus, anecdotally I would propose that when we do see anaplastic endometrial carcinoma in a young woman under the age of 40, the prognosis would not be as good as that for a grade III lesion in a patient over 40.

Dr. Silverberg: I think it is well established in the literature that anaplastic lesions are not more dangerous in young patients than in older patients, as established in several series. The reason that the general survival of endometrial carcinoma in young women is very good is that the great majority of the cases are well-differentiated tumors. We have shown that both in women under age 40 taking oral contraceptives and in those not taking them, the great majority of the lesions are well-differentiated tumors, usually with little or no myometrial invasion, so these patients do very well. When we reviewed the literature and looked at several large series of young patients with endometrial carcinoma, we were able to find a total mortality rate of 7.2%. In other words, the cure rate was 93% for endometrial carcinomas in patients under 40 years of age. The patients who died were almost always predictable cases, in accord with our Armed Forces Institute of Pathology data. In almost every case, you could have predicted that the young woman would die on the basis of the fact that she had an anaplastic tumor, a mixed carcinoma, a clear-cell carcinoma, or obvious deep myometrial invasion and/or spread outside the uterus at the time of hysterectomy. Every patient in whom none of these factors existed survived, without exception.

Dr. Morris: Dr. Major, you just said that the anaplastic tumor in the young patient is worse than the same tumor in the older patient. Actually, our experience has been that younger patients do better, but I don't know that we've conducted a careful classification of the very anaplastic tumors to make a comparison. Most women who are age 70 or 80 are not expected to live 5 years anyway, and the younger patient is a better surgical risk, and I can do more for her.

Dr. Silverberg: Do you have any comment on that, Dr. Sommers?

Dr. Sommers: There is an uncommon variety of endometrial carcinoma developing before or at age 30 in the woman who has had trouble from menarche on, probably because she has never or rarely ovulated. She has had serial curettages that revealed cystic and, then more progressively, dysplastic endometrium, and she may or may not have been treated with hormones of various kinds, or with radiation in the old days, to attempt to control the bleeding. When her tumor finally develops, it is anaplastic, and those women are represented in the few cases already mentioned.

Dr. Silverberg: Any questions from the audience?

Question: What is the present status of understanding on the relation of Depo-Provera to cervical cancer?

Dr. Stadel: The Food and Drug Administration was prepared to conditionally approve Depo-Provera for marketing after review of the data on its relationship to cervical carcinoma. A series of political hearings eventually led to a suspension of this action, which is the current status on this issue. The review of the data is such that it is not possible to determine whether Depo-Provera increases, decreases, or does not alter the risk of cervical dysplasia or carcinoma in situ. Everyone involved in the review felt that these questions might be resolved by a properly controlled study. However, the available data were a series from an exposed group of women, which were then controlled to various sets of figures from either the literature or from national survey statistics. The risk among the exposed women fits into the spectrum of possibilities that could be expected in a population depending on the presence or absence of other known risk factors. One cannot conclude that there is a clear red warning sign. However, the issue became extremely sensitive politically.

Question: What about the animal studies on breast tumors?

Dr. Stadel: I don't know of any human data on the issue. There is concern from studies on beagles, and there is concern about the studies on beagles. There is little doubt that DMPA causes nodules in beagle breasts, but the degree to which one wants to consider that a cautionary finding for its use in humans, the degree to which one makes that jump of faith, varies widely, depending on who one is in the current setting. There are no human data concerning this issue.

Question: Dr. Silverberg, another paper was recently published or submitted for publication at a similar time as your initial paper on Oracon in which the author also found that endometrial biopsies of patients taking Oracon had adenomatous hyperplasia. What do you think is the significance of that finding?

Dr. Silverberg: Dr. Lyon in Minneapolis reported four cases of endometrial carcinoma in women taking Oracon about the same time we reported our first 21 cases. Three of his four patients were over age 40, and the other one was under 40 and was included in our series because he had sent us that case for review. He subsequently reported a series of endometrial biopsies in 12 women taking Oracon, in whom he found adenomatous hyperplasia in seven, a very high prevalence (Lyon FA, Frisch MJ: Obstet Gynecol **47:**639, 1976). However, this has not been our experience, as I mentioned before. We reviewed some material from Dr. Jack L. Adams in Albuquerque, who had a large number of women taking Oracon, and he sent us Vabra aspirates from 37 of them. Four specimens were inadequate, and of the other 33, we found only four (12.1%) that we thought were significantly hyperplastic; the rest were mostly proliferative endometrium. This is usually what you find in women taking Oracon: we found that the incidence of hyperplasia was much lower than that reported in Dr. Lyon's series. Dr. Kreutner (Kreutner A, Johnson D, Williamson HO: Fertil Steril **70:**905, 1976) in South Carolina has also reviewed 111 biopsies, more than Dr. Lyon and us put together, in asymptomatic women who were taking Oracon over a long period of time, and his incidence of hyperplasia was also quite low (13.5%), which again would lead me to think that if you are trying to put together a population-based denominator, the actual risk is probably fairly low. However, even an incidence of hyperplasia of 12 or 13% seems high in a population of young, previously fertile women.

I might mention, talking about the political atmosphere of the hearings, that it is important to realize that these decisions are not made in a political vacuum. Dr. Sommers mentioned the fact that he was at the FDA hearing at which one of Ralph Nader's people talked about drug companies making money and killing millions of women with endometrial carcinoma. The other side of the spectrum was the lady, presumably postmenopausal, who kept getting up every time a man made a statement and saying, "you have never had a hot flash," and "you can't take our estrogens away from us." The decisions are made in the political arena in which both of these extreme viewpoints were being discussed.

Question: Are there any data about hydroxyprogesterone causing breast tumors, benign or malignant, in humans?

Dr. Stadel: Our contraceptive development branch has studies of both danizol and sublingual methyltestosterone in progress, but I do not know whether they are currently studying DMPA as a male contraceptive.

Vaginal and Cervical Pathology Associated With Prenatal Exposure to Diethylstilbestrol

Stanley J. Robboy, M.D.

Jaime Prat, M.D.

William R. Welch, M.D.

In 1971, intrauterine exposure to diethylstilbestrol (DES) was linked to the rare development of clear-cell adenocarcinoma of the vagina and was subsequently shown to be related to clear-cell adenocarcinoma of the cervix, nonneoplastic abnormalities of the lower genital tract in the female (vaginal adenosis, cervical ectropion, vaginal and cervical ridges) and, more recently, to anomalies of the epididymis and testis in the male. This chapter will review the pathologic findings in DES-exposed subjects, new observations and recent advances, and the current status of attempts to develop animal models.

CLEAR-CELL ADENOCARCINOMA

On the basis of data from more than 330 cases in the Registry of Clear-cell Adenocarcinoma of the Genital Tract in Young Females accumulated by 1977, most patients with clear-cell adenocarcinoma of the vagina or cervix were found to be born in the United States (20, 40); a few have been reported from Mexico, Canada, Europe, Australia, and Africa. The average age of the patients at the time of diagnosis has been 19 years. Although an occasional patient has been as young as 7 years of age, almost all have been over the age of 14 years; the oldest was 28. Approximately 65% of the patients had documented exposure in utero

Supported in part by National Institutes of Health Contract NO1-CN-45157 and Biomedical Research Support Grant 5-S07-RR05486-15 to the Massachusetts General Hospital and by American Cancer Society Junior Faculty Fellowship (J.P. and W.R.W.) and Grant PDT-89.

to DES; another 10% were exposed to some form of medication for high-risk pregnancy, but in these cases, the prenatal records were not available for examination. The majority of the patients with negative histories had tumors that were cervical in origin, a finding consistent with the observation that clear-cell adenocarcinoma of the cervix in young women was a well-recognized entity prior to the DES era, whereas clear-cell adenocarcinoma of the vagina was exceedingly rare. In all of the cases in which detailed information has been available, it was found that the drug had been administered prior to the 18th week of gestation. It is estimated at the present time that the tumor develops in 0.014–0.14% of exposed females (18).

Initially, most patients were examined because of vaginal bleeding or discharge, but, more recently, asymptomatic tumors have been detected as more young women have begun to seek examination only because of known exposure.

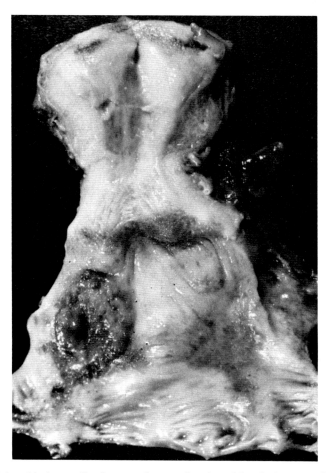

Figure 1. Polypoid clear-cell adenocarcinoma, bordered by dark zone of adenosis, lies on anterior vaginal wall; another patch of adenosis occupies posterior wall (*lower right*). The vaginal adenosis and extensive ectropion of cervix appeared red in fresh state. (By permission of *Cancer* **25:**745, 1970.)

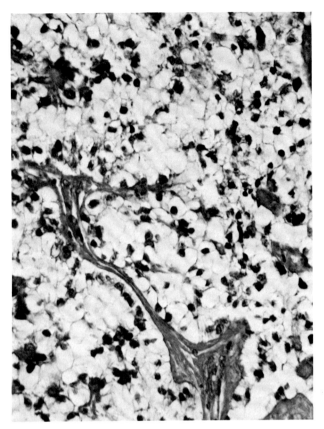

Figure 2. Clear-cell adenocarcinoma. Clear-cell pattern of tumor, which resembles clear-cell carcinoma of ovary and endometrium. Hematoxylin and eosin; ×300. (By permission of *Annals of Clinical Laboratory Science* **4:**222, 1974.)

Careful inspection and palpation of the entire cervix and vagina together with iodine staining of the mucosa have played an important role in the detection of the neoplasm, especially when it is small, confined to the lamina propria, and covered by intact normal or metaplastic squamous epithelium.

The tumor may involve any portion of the vagina and/or cervix. Approximately 60% of lesions have been confined to the vagina; the remainder have been limited to the cervix or have involved both the cervix and vagina. Most of the vaginal tumors arose on the anterior wall, usually in the upper third, a location that corresponds to the most frequent site of adenosis. The lateral and posterior walls and, occasionally, the middle and lower third of the vagina have also been involved.

The smallest tumor has been 3 mm in greatest diameter, and the largest was more than 10 cm. Most are polypoid and nodular (Figure 1), but some are flat or ulcerated, with a granular or indurated surface. Occasionally, a tumor may appear clinically to be multicentric, but submucosal continuity between these foci has been observed microscopically in some of these cases. "Kissing lesions" on the

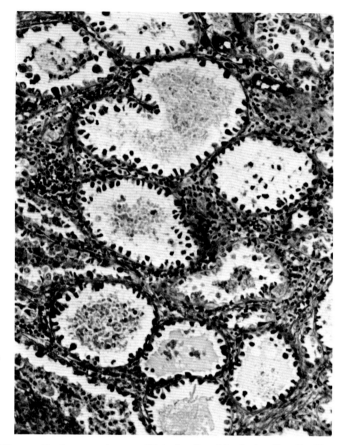

Figure 3. Clear-cell adenocarcinoma. Tubules lined by hobnail cells. Hematoxylin and eosin; ×180. (By permission of *Annals of Clinical Laboratory Science* **4:**222, 1974.)

wall opposite the main tumor have also rarely been seen. Although the majority of cancers are superficial and invade only a few millimeters into the vaginal or cervical wall, microscopic examination has disclosed that some of them have penetrated more deeply or extended more centrifugally than can be ascertained by gross examination alone (50).

By light and electron microscopy, the clear-cell adenocarcinoma associated with DES exposure is identical to the clear-cell adenocarcinomas of the ovary and endometrium, which occur sporadically in older women (34, 39, 45). A characteristic pattern, for which the tumor is named, consists of solid sheets of clear cells (Figure 2); for many years, this pattern was considered the diagnostic sine qua non of the neoplasm. In hematoxylin and eosin-stained sections, the clear appearance of the cytoplasm is due to the dissolution of glycogen as the tissue specimen is prepared for microscopic examination. With appropriate fixation and staining methods, intracytoplasmic glycogen can be demonstrated. The second and most frequent pattern is characterized by tubules and cysts lined by "hobnail" cells (Figure 3), flat cells, or by cells that resemble to various degrees

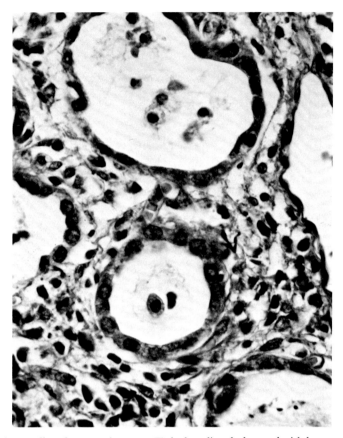

Figure 4. Clear-cell adenocarcinoma. Tubules lined by cuboidal neoplastic cells. Hematoxylin and eosin; ×490.

the epithelium of the mullerian tract but that lack features so distinctive as to warrant a special designation (Figure 4). The hobnail cell is characterized by a bulbous nucleus that protrudes into the lumen beyond the apparent cytoplasmic limits of the cell. Flat cells often appear deceptively innocuous; when only this type of epithelium is observed, for example, in a small biopsy, it may be very difficult to differentiate the tumor from adenosis, which is benign. Other patterns encountered include complex papillae (Figure 5) and trabeculae. In any of the above patterns, the lumen may contain mucus; except in rare instances, the cytoplasm is mucin-free.

The cells of clear-cell adenocarcinoma can be detected cytologically, and, occasionally, a suspicious or positive smear may provide the first indication of an asymptomatic tumor (48). With the use of circumferential vaginal and cervical scrapes and endocervical aspirations, a high percentage of tumors should probably be detected. The tumor cells often resemble large endocervical cells (Figure 6) but vary greatly and may appear even as undifferentiated carcinoma. False-negative results in 20% of cases are due to the difficulty in distinguishing tumor cells from endocervical cells, the heavy overlay of polymorphonuclear leuko-

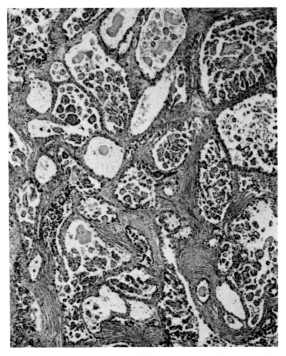

Figure 5. Clear-cell adenocarcinoma, papillary pattern. Hematoxylin and eosin; ×140. (From *Pathology of the Female Genital Tract* by permission of Springer-Verlag.)

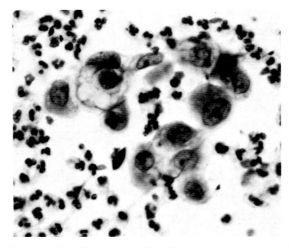

Figure 6. Vaginal smear in which clear-cell adenocarcinoma resembles large atypical endocervical cells. Papanicolaou stain; ×540.

cytes, and the possibility that some of the exposed neoplasms may not shed cells. Other causes of negative results are the occasional confinement of the tumor to the lamina propria and the fact that prior diagnostic biopsies have sometimes resulted in excision of all of the tumor.

The tumor spreads locally and also metastasizes via lymphatics and blood vessels. Approximately one sixth of tumors that are confined clinically to the vagina or cervix (stage I) metastasize to the pelvic lymph nodes. The frequency of nodal involvement reaches approximately 50% when only stage II tumors are considered. The clear-cell cancer extends outside the abdominal cavity more frequently than does squamous cell carcinoma that arises in the same organs. This distinction is illustrated by the fact that the sites of one third of the first recurrences of clear-cell carcinomas are in the supraclavicular lymph nodes and lungs, whereas these organs are involved in less than 10% of the recurrences of squamous cell carcinoma (36).

Although many patients have been followed for several years, sufficient data have not yet been accumulated for definitive recommendations regarding the optimal form of therapy. Since recurrences have been detected in approximately 25% of cases, it is apparent, however, that clear-cell carcinoma can be aggressive. Although most recurrences occurred within the first 2 years after excision of the primary tumor, a few have appeared more than 5 years later. Factors associated with a worse prognosis are the presence of symptoms at the time the tumor was first detected and local excision, which cannot be guaranteed to remove the tumor (20, 36). Large-size and/or deep invasion into the wall often are associated with a poor prognosis, but small or superficial tumors may also recur. The number of mitoses may be of some help to gauge prognosis, and these phenomena are encountered more often in cervical than vaginal tumors and more often in younger than older patients. Most of the patients with recurrences have died.

NONNEOPLASTIC ANOMALIES

Several nonneoplastic anomalies of the vagina and cervix have been associated with DES exposure, all of which occur far more frequently than does clear-cell adenocarcinoma. These anomalies include vaginal adenosis, cervical ectropion, and vaginal and cervical ridges; the latter has been given such descriptive designations as hoods, collars, rims, cock's combs, and pseudopolyps (Figure 7) (19, 43). Deformities of the uterine corpus, such as T-shaped appearance of the cavity, constricting bands in the cavity, hypoplasia, and, rarely, synechiae, have been observed with hysterosalpingographic studies (24), but these findings have not been confirmed by gross pathologic studies, and their physiologic significance has not yet been ascertained. Rare congenital anomalies of the cardiovascular system have also been reported (16) but have been associated with both steroidal and nonsteroidal estrogens and progestogens.

Vaginal adenosis, that is, the presence of glandular epithelium or its secretory products in the vagina, is a common finding in the DES-exposed female. In the pre-DES era, vaginal adenosis was a medical rarity that occurred occasionally in

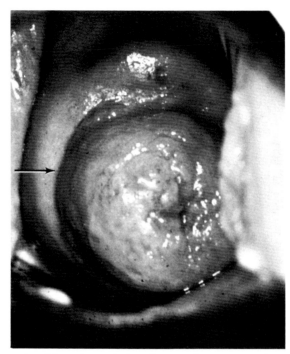

Figure 7. Concentric ridge (arrow) in the cervix creates the appearance of a "pseudopolyp" in the center of which is the external os. A circular fold gives the appearance of a hood covering the cervix. (By permission of *Journal of Reproductive Medicine* **15**:13, 1975.)

women, usually in their 30s or 40s. Not surprisingly, it was also found more frequently in autopsy studies in which the vagina was extensively sampled microscopically (25, 42). In 3–5% of fetuses and infants, colposcopic and pathologic examination at the time of autopsy have revealed that the squamocolumnar junction lies in the vaginal fornix rather than in the cervix (33). Adenosis should be suspected clinically when the vaginal mucosa contains red granular spots or patches (Figure 1), does not stain with an iodine solution (Figure 8), or is colposcopically abnormal (19). In 75% of cases, adenosis involves the upper half of the anterior vaginal wall; the anterior wall only is involved in 55% of cases, the posterior wall only in 10%, and the lateral wall only in 4% (32). Although the upper half of the vagina is usually involved, the adenosis is confined to the lower half in 9% and near the hymen in 2% of cases.

The glandular epithelium in most cases of vaginal adenosis consists of mucinous columnar cells, which by light (14, 32, 39) or electron microscopy (11) resemble those of the normal endocervical mucosa (Figure 9). Dark or light cells, which are often ciliated, are similar to the lining of the normal fallopian tube or the endometrium and are found in less than one third of cases of adenosis (Figure 9). In approximately 10% of cases, both types of epithelia are encountered in separate glands within the same biopsy specimen or, occasionally, even within a single gland. In an occasional biopsy specimen from an area in the distal vagina or in other areas in which the vaginal mucosa stains normally with

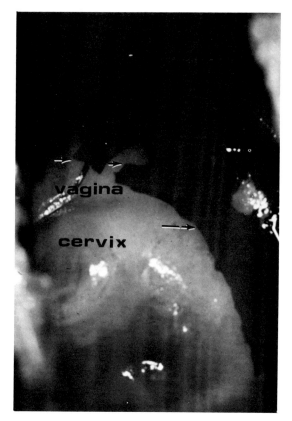

Figure 8. Abnormal Schiller stain in which aglycogenated (nonstaining) areas in both the vagina and the cervix appear white in the photograph and represent the so-called transformation zone. The glycogenated vaginal epithelium stains black. Arrows demarcate the staining from the nonstaining areas. (By permission of *Journal of Reproductive Medicine* **15:**13, 1975.)

iodine, the adenosis may appear as tiny glands lined by cells without distinctive cytoplasmic features and located at the interface of the squamous mucosa and lamina propria (Figure 10).

   In the majority of biopsy specimens, the adenosis is replaced to various degrees by metaplastic squamous cells (Figure 11), suggesting that the adenosis heals as a result of squamous metaplasia, beginning as reserve cell proliferation and progressing through the stages of immature and mature squamous metaplasia. After the metaplastic squamous epithelium becomes filled with glycogen, it is indistinguishable from the normal squamous epithelium. In part, the frequency and extent of squamous metaplasia are related to age of the patient. The relative percentages of columnar cells and metaplastic squamous cells in biopsies from young patients are approximately 90 and 10%, respectively, with the relative percentage of columnar cells declining to less than 20% and that of metaplastic squamous cells rising to more than 80% in subjects 30 years and older (32). Cytologic smears also reflect quantitatively these changes. During the course of replacement of glands by metaplastic squamous epithelium, the glan-

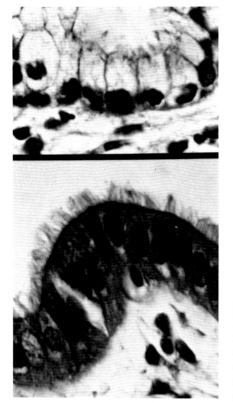

Figure 9. Glandular epithelium of adenosis. Mucinous epithelium (*top*) resembles the normal endocervical mucosa. Hematoxylin and eosin; ×775. Ciliated epithelium (*bottom*) with dark cytoplasm resembles the normal lining of the tube or endometrium. Hematoxylin and eosin; ×890.

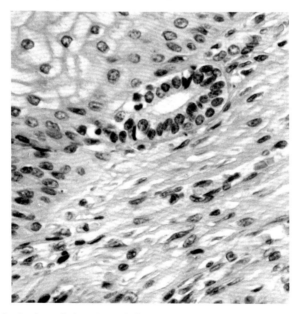

Figure 10. Vaginal adenosis in 28-week fetus. Adenosis in infants, in the distal portion of the vagina, or in areas in which the mucosa stains normally with iodine, often appears immature, without signs of cytoplasmic differentiation. Hematoxylin and eosin; ×400. (By permission of *Human Pathology* **5**:265, 1974.)

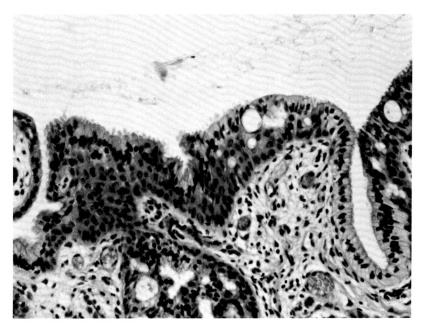

Figure 11. Vaginal adenosis with mucinous columnar epithelium lying on the surface of metaplastic squamous epithelium (*center* and *left*). To the right, the mucinous epithelium appears to line the neck of a gland in the lamina propria. Hematoxylin and eosin; ×250. (By permission of *Journal of Reproductive Medicine* **15**:13, 1975.)

dular epithelium becomes reduced in amount and may appear in the form of intercellular pools of mucin in which the cells that line the pool are flattened mucinous cells (Figure 12). A final vestige consists of intracellular droplets of mucin in immature metaplastic squamous cells (39). Glands and their openings to the surface, when completely replaced by squamous epithelium, appear in the lamina propria as squamous pegs; serial sections reveal that they are continuous with the metaplastic squamous epithelium covering the surface of the vagina (14, 39).

Depending on the population of subjects examined, the frequency of adenosis, abnormal colposcopic findings, and areas that fail to stain with iodine in the vagina vary from 33 to more than 90% of patients. The paucity or lack of glycogen in the metaplastic squamous epithelium accounts for the abnormal iodine stain (2, 14, 19), while the increased vascularity, tortuous arrangement of the vessels that surround the pegs in the lamina propria, and the chronic inflammatory infiltrate are responsible for the atypical colposcopic patterns, such as mosaicism and punctation, seen so often in this condition. Hyperkeratosis accounts for the colposcopic finding of leukoplakia (51).

Cervical ectropion, that is, the presence of glandular epithelium or its secretory products in the cervical portio, occurs in nearly all exposed females and is probably closely related to adenosis. Although most of the features described for adenosis are applicable to ectropion, several observations suggest that these processes may differ in part, and therefore we prefer to consider them sepa-

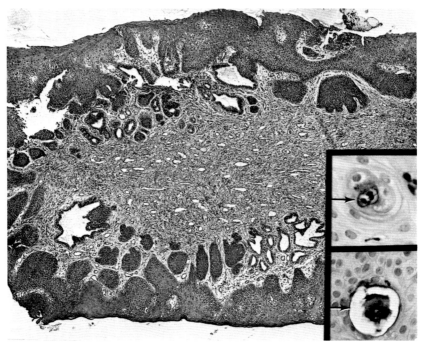

Figure 12. Vaginal adenosis in the lamina propria of the vagina. Metaplastic squamous cells line the surface of the vagina and the squamous pegs continuous with it. Hematoxylin and eosin; ×43. *Insets:* Mucinous droplets (*upper*) and pools (*lower*) in metaplastic squamous epithelium (mucicarmine stain, ×350 and ×240, respectively). (By permission of *Obstetrics and Gynecology* **48:**511, 1976.)

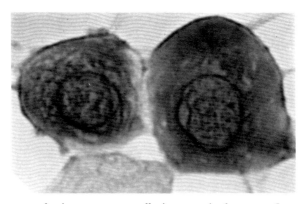

Figure 13. Two metaplastic squamous cells in a vaginal scrape from a patient with vaginal adenosis. Papanicolaou stain; ×1890. (By permission of *Journal of Reproductive Medicine* **15:**13, 1975.)

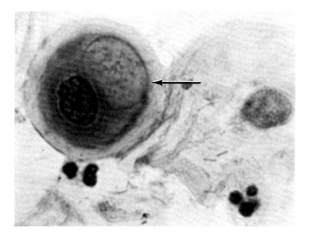

Figure 14. Metaplastic squamous cell with a mucin droplet (arrow) in a vaginal scrape from a patient with vaginal adenosis. Papanicolaou stain; ×1445. (By permission of *Journal of Reproductive Medicine* **15:**13, 1975.)

rately for the purposes of this chapter. First, ciliated cells, which have been identified frequently in the vagina, are rare in the cervix (39). Second, adenosis most often occurs in the form of glands in the lamina propria, whereas in ectropion, the glandular epithelium commonly lines the surface of the cervix. Until the embryologic etiologies of these abnormalities are understood and their natural history and responses to therapy are established, we believe that separation of adenosis and ectropion will permit more accurate comparison of their features from one institution to another.

Cytologic studies, in addition to their usefulness in the detection of malignancy, are also helpful in the detection of adenosis and in raising the suspicion that the individual might have been exposed in utero to DES. In smears obtained by scraping the middle and upper thirds of the entire circumference of the vagina, columnar cells with mucinous cytoplasm or metaplastic squamous cells have been found in more than 34% of cases; these cells are found in 54% of scrapes of the exocervix (Figure 13) (35). An occasional metaplastic cell may contain an intracytoplasmic droplet of mucin (Figure 14). Other investigators have recorded even higher percentages (up to 78% in the vagina) (4, 15, 32). Although these cells are absent in vaginal samples from control subjects, one must always be careful to exclude the possibility that the spatula used to obtain the vaginal smear has touched an ectropion of the cervix and thereby become contaminated.

COMPLICATIONS OF ADENOSIS AND ECTROPION

The glandular epithelium of adenosis and ectropion and the metaplastic squamous epithelium that develops as a physiologic reaction to these glandular cell types are susceptible to the same range of pathologic changes that have been encountered in the cervix of the nonexposed female.

Atypical Adenosis

The glandular epithelium of adenosis is believed to provide the bed from which the clear-cell adenocarcinoma arises, possibly through the transitional state of atypical adenosis. Atypical adenosis, usually in the form of one or a few glands with cellular stratification, nuclear pleomorphism, and hyperchromasia and prominent nucleoli, has been identified near the periphery of several carcinomas (Figure 15) (40). Atypical glands have also been identified in approximately 0.5% of cervical and vaginal smears as cells with nuclei that are larger and more irregular in outline than those seen in normal endocervical cells or the cells that line the glands of the adenosis (35). The frequent finding of the tuboendometrial type of glandular cells and the rarity of the mucinous type of cells that surround the tumors, in addition to the occurrence in older women of clear-cell adenocarcinomas arising in the endometrium where mucinous cells are usually absent, have suggested that the tuboendometrial type of cell may be the one from which the clear-cell adenocarcinoma arises.

Dysplasia

It has been predicted that squamous cell neoplasia will develop with increasing frequency in the DES-exposed population (27). In the unexposed female, cervical ectropion heals as a result of the formation of squamous metaplasia, which eventually becomes mature and indistinguishable from normal squamous

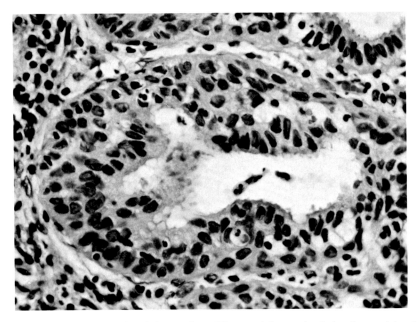

Figure 15. Atypical adenosis of the vagina. The nuclei vary both in size and in shape, and the cells are stratified. Hematoxylin and eosin; ×500. (From *Pathology of the Female Genital Tract* by permission of Springer-Verlag.)

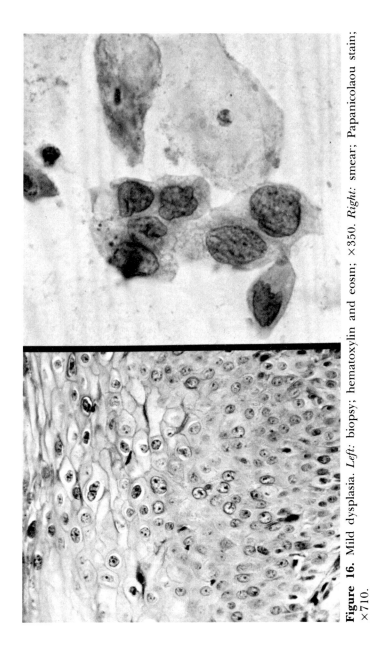

Figure 16. Mild dysplasia. *Left*: biopsy; hematoxylin and eosin; ×350. *Right*: smear; Papanicolaou stain; ×710.

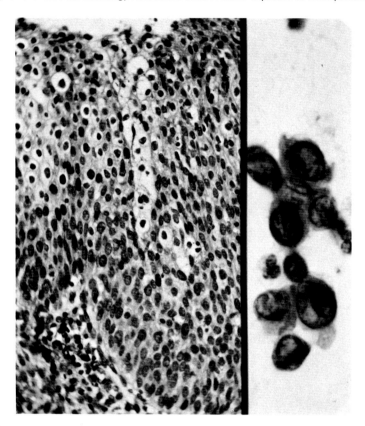

Figure 17. Severe dysplasia. *Left:* biopsy; hematoxylin and eosin; ×290. *Right:* smear; Papanicolaou stain; ×710.

epithelium. Occasionally, immature metaplastic epithelium may not differentiate normally but, instead, evolve into dysplasia, carcinoma in situ (CIS), or squamous cell carcinoma. In 1974, the finding of squamous cell dysplasia in a small number of exposed subjects led investigators to speculate that the incidence of in situ and invasive squamous cell carcinoma of the lower genital tract would rise greatly as the exposed population reaches the peak ages at which these lesions are encountered in the cervix of unexposed women (47). This prediction has precipitated a controversy regarding the frequency of dysplasia and CIS in exposed females and the validity of the prediction itself (38). Of 1424 women followed at the Massachusetts General Hospital since 1971, the prevalence of dysplasia has been 2.1% and the incidence 0.85/100 person-years of follow-up (37). The dysplasia was almost always mild and was slightly more frequent in the cervix than in the vagina (Figure 16). Severe dysplasia and CIS were encountered only in subjects specifically referred because of that abnormality (Figure 17). The frequency of dysplasia was lowest when the patients were identified through a review of prenatal records, was intermediate when they were referred by other physicians because of a known exposure to DES, and was highest in women who themselves requested examination (26). The most common problem in the diagnosis of squamous cell neoplasia has been the misinterpretation of immature squamous metaplasia for dysplasia. Immature squamous metaplasia is characterized by an

increased cellularity, minimal differentiation of the cytoplasm, and the occasional presence of mitoses above the basal layer; however, the nuclei are not
hyperchromatic and vary little in size and shape, and abnormal forms are not
encountered. On the basis of established criteria, we would reclassify some of the
published cases illustrated as carcinoma in situ and dysplasia in those series with
the unusually high rates of precancerous changes (27) as falling in a range from
immature squamous metaplasia to moderate dysplasia. Since discordance between cytology and biopsy was commonplace in the detection and follow-up of
dysplasia, especially in the milder forms (37), the frequency of dysplasia is
therefore influenced by whether the patients are screened by cytology alone,
biopsy alone, or both. Other factors that affect the prevalence rate of dysplasia
include the sexual activity of the population studied and the misinterpretation of
atypical columnar cells as dysplastic squamous cells.

Microglandular Hyperplasia

Microglandular hyperplasia is a benign, tumor-like condition, usually associated
with long-term ingestion of oral contraceptive agents and occasionally with
pregnancy. At the time this lesion was first described in the cervix in 1967, it was
emphasized that it could be easily confused with adenocarcinoma. Recently,
eight cases of microglandular hyperplasia have been reported that arose in foci
of adenosis in the vagina of young females, five of whom had been exposed
prenatally to DES (41); each of these lesions had been misinterpreted initially as
clear-cell adenocarcinoma. Grossly, the lesion is soft, tan-yellow, and usually
flat to granular. Occasionally, it may be cauliflower-like or multicentric (Figure
18). On microscopic examination, myriads of tiny glands that are devoid of

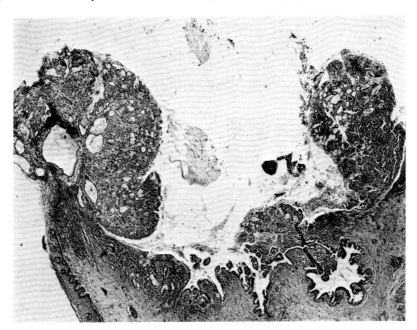

Figure 18. Microglandular hyperplasia. Edges of polypoid mass in vagina where the
empty space (*center*) is the biopsy site. At the base is a focus of adenosis. Hematoxylin and
eosin; ×23. (By permission of *Obstetrics and Gynecology* **49:**430, 1977.)

intervening stroma are observed to be arranged in a reticular pattern (Figure 19). The nuclei of the cells that line the glands are uniform in size and shape and have finely dispersed chromatin. The glandular lumina contain mucin and an acute inflammatory cell infiltrate; intracellular mucin is variable. The presence of extensive nests of metaplastic squamous cells with filmy eosinophilic cytoplasm may make the lesion especially difficult to distinguish from the solid pattern of clear-cell carcinoma. The clue to the proper diagnosis is the presence of clefts lined by mucinous epithelium that course through the metaplastic squamous epithelium. The fact that the microglands have been observed in continuity with the clefts suggests that the former result from budding and arborization of the mucinous epithelium of the type that lines the normal endocervix and also constitutes one type of vaginal adenosis. Microglandular hyperplasia has not been observed to arise from the type of adenosis characterized by an epithelium that resembles the endometrium or fallopian tube. The lesion is generally reversed by discontinuance of oral contraceptive medication.

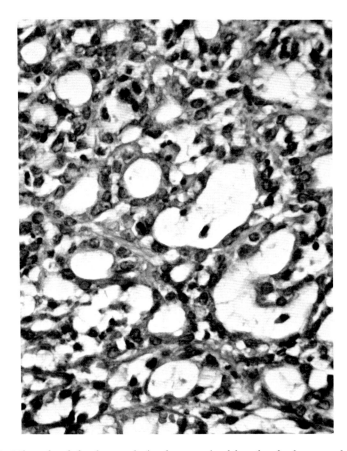

Figure 19. Microglandular hyperplasia characterized by glands that are closely packed and separated by little or no stroma. The nuclei are uniform and have relatively fine, evenly dispersed chromatin. Hematoxylin and eosin; ×490. (By permission of *Obstetrics and Gynecology* **49:**430, 1977.)

REPRODUCTION

Recent preliminary data suggest that reproductive abnormalities may occur more frequently in DES-exposed females than in nonexposed individuals. Female offspring of mothers who participated in a double-blind, placebo-controlled investigation during 1951–2 had differences in their frequency and irregularity of menstruation, duration of flow, and pregnancy history (4). Oligomenorrhea was the most common menstrual irregularity, occurring in 18% of exposed and 10% of nonexposed females. The menstrual flow lasted 1–4 days in 60% of exposed females, in contrast to 5–7 days in 55% of controls. Although only 18% of exposed women had been pregnant, as opposed to 33% of controls, the inability to achieve pregnancy, if desired, was similar in both groups. In mice treated prenatally with DES, reproductive capacity was impaired and appeared to be dose related. The number of births fell to less than 4% of controls as the dosage reached 5% of the average daily amount given to pregnant women therapeutically (28).

EMBRYOLOGY AND ANIMAL EXPERIMENTATION

It is generally agreed that clear-cell adenocarcinoma, vaginal adenosis, and cervical ectropion are of mullerian origin. In earlier years, it was believed that the clear-cell cancer, previously known as "mesonephroma," arose from the mesonephric ducts. Such an origin is at best very rare, because extensive sectioning of vaginas in the Registry has not disclosed a single instance in which the neoplasm arose topographically in relation to the mesonephric ducts. Furthermore, the mesonephric ducts are found deep in the lateral wall of the vagina and cervix, whereas most clear-cell cancers arise superficially on the anterior wall in areas where adenosis is also present. Further support for this hypothesis is provided by the fact that the clear-cell carcinoma that occurs in the endometrium originates from the endometrium itself, which is mullerian in origin, and the clear-cell carcinoma that occurs in the ovary is frequently associated with endometriosis.

Although it is also agreed that the vagina has an ancestry in both mullerian duct and urogenital sinus tissues, the exact contribution of each is not clear nor is the mechanism by which prenatal exposure to DES distorts the developing vagina and the embryonic mullerian epithelium develops into tumor. Several investigators have suggested that the cranial 60% of the vagina is of mullerian origin and that the caudal 40% arises from the urogenital sinus (6). This postulate, however, is not consistent with the observation that both clear-cell carcinoma and adenosis, which are believed to be mullerian in origin, may be confined to the lower third of the vagina or even the hymen (20, 32). Other investigators have suggested that the vaginal epithelium in the developing fetus is mullerian in origin but, subsequently, is replaced by a squamous cell epithelium that is entirely urogenital sinus in origin. On the basis of studies in nonexposed individuals with congenital anomalies of the vagina, we favor the hypothesis that the development of the human vagina is best explained by the latter theory (49). After the mullerian ducts extend caudally during early fetal life to the level of the future hymen, they fuse and form a muscular scaffold on which the squamous cells, which derive from the urogenital sinus, invade from below, replacing completely the mullerian mucosa up to the level of the external os of the cervical canal. Since this entire process begins sometime after the fourth or fifth week of intrauterine life and is not complete until sometime after the 20th week of pregnancy, it is possible that DES may act to inhibit the replacement of the mullerian epithelium by squamous epithelium or, possibly, to stimulate the persistence of the mullerian epithelium in the vagina. The residual mullerian epithelium results in adenosis and may give rise to clear-cell adenocarcinoma. If the surrounding mesodermal stroma from which the muscular walls of the vagina, cervix, and uterus derive is affected, one might also expect to see the ridges, partial strictures, obliterations, fish-mouth deformities of the cervix, and uterine abnormalities that have been described in the DES-exposed female.

Several animal species have been utilized in recent years in an attempt to develop an animal model in which adenosis and clear-cell cancer will develop. In at least three different laboratories (3, 12, 52), a condition that resembles adenosis of the vagina has been produced in mice treated neonatally with a variety of different estrogens, including DES and synthetic estrogenic compounds. Unlike the human, in whom the glandular epithelium of adenosis may be composed of cells with intracellular mucin or dark cytoplasm, often with cilia, the glands in the mouse appear relatively immature, lacking distinctive cytoplasmic features (Figure 20). Jones and Bern have demonstrated that the adenosis in animals may proliferate markedly over long periods of time and resemble a neoplastic growth, with both squamous and glandular components

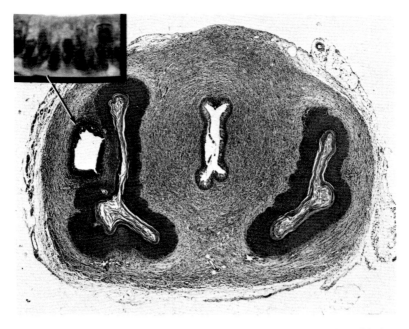

Figure 20. Vaginal adenosis (arrow) in fornix of mouse exposed at birth to DES. Hematoxylin and eosin; ×35. *Inset:* Glandular epithelium in adenosis. Hematoxylin and eosin; ×690. (Courtesy of Dr. Linda Plapinger, The Rockefeller University.)

(21). Although well differentiated, it is transplantable and grows autonomously. This tumor, however, does not contain clear cells, and it is not certain whether it is analogous to that which occurs in humans.

ANOMALIES IN MALES

Although there is no known association at present between DES exposure and neoplasia in males, nonmalignant anomalies have been reported and have included epididymal cysts, abnormalities of the penile urethra, and small testes. In a follow-up study of mothers and controls who were treated with DES and a placebo, respectively, in the early 1950s, abnormalities were found in 25% of 163 DES-exposed male offspring, in contrast to 6% of 168 control offspring (4). The quality of semen was "severely pathologic" in 28% of the exposed group, compared to zero in the controls. In a second study, penile stenosis or hypospadias was found in 4.4% of exposed subjects but in no controls (17). In addition, three of 11 of the exposed group who were examined had undescended testes (5). In one of the few case reports on adverse effects of prenatal exposure to DES published before 1971, when DES was linked to clear-cell adenocarcinoma, a male pseudohermaphrodite was born with hypospadias; the testes were apparently devoid of germ cells (23). Experimentally, 60% of male mice exposed prenatally to DES are sterile and have testicular anomalies (29). Nodular enlargement of the seminal vesicle and prostate have also been observed (28). The implications of these findings for reproductive capacity in man will not be known until further follow-up data are available.

THE FUTURE

Investigations in progress are employing numerous different approaches. Clinical studies of the behavior of the tumor continue in several centers throughout the United States. Large-scale clinical projects have begun to study the natural history of adenosis and to determine the most cost-effective method of examining the DES-exposed population (1). In the search for tumor markers, cathepsin levels in blood have been found to be elevated in patients with either adenosis or adenocarcinoma (33). The psychologic effects on patients of knowledge of their exposure (44) and the potential risks to women who are pregnant while continuing to consume meats of animals in which DES was used as feed (22) are currently under investigation.

Animal studies have focused on the mechanisms of action of DES. What is the fate of DES when given to pregnant mothers? Several studies have indicated that DES localizes preferentially in the reproductive organs of the fetus (30, 31, 46). Cunha et al. have examined factors that control the development of the reproductive organs, in particular, the interrelations among the stroma of the embryonic gonadal ridge and those of the developing mullerian and wolffian ductal structures (7–10). Their studies in the mouse have already established the fact that the stroma of the uterus and of the vagina play an active role in the formation of these organs and that they act as inducers to the types of epithelium that ultimately are characteristic in the adult.

In summary, much has been learned since 1971 about the biology of prenatal exposure to DES. The many approaches used in current investigations promise rapid expansion of knowledge about many facets of this disorder in the future.

REFERENCES

1. Anon: Exposure in utero to diethylstilbestrol and related synthetic hormones. Association with vaginal and cervical cancers and other abnormalities. J Amer Med Ass **236:**1107, 1976.

2. Antonioli DA, Burke L: Vaginal adenosis. Analysis of 325 biopsy specimens from 100 patients. Amer J Clin Pathol **64:**625, 1975.

3. Bern HA, Jones LA, Mills KT: Use of the neonatal mouse in studying long-term effects of early exposure to hormones and other agents. J Toxicol Environ Health **1:**103, 1976.

4. Bibbo M, Gill WB, Azizi F, et al: Follow-up study of male and female offspring of DES-exposed mothers. Obstet Gynecol **49:**1, 1977.

5. Cosgrove M, Benton B, Henderson B: Male genitourinary abnormalities and maternal diethylstilbestrol. J Urol **117:**220, 1977.

6. Cunha GR: The dual origin of vaginal epithelium. Amer J Anat **143:**387, 1975.

7. Cunha GR: Alterations in the developmental properties of stroma during the development of the urogenital ridge into ductus deferens and uterus in embryonic and neonatal mice. J Exp Zool **197:**375, 1976.

8. Cunha GR: Epthelial-stromal interactions in development of the urogenital tract. Int Rev Cytol **47:**137, 1976.

9. Cunha GR: Stromal induction and specification of morphogenesis and cytodifferentiation of the epithelia of the mullerian ducts and urogenital sinus during development of the uterus and vagina in mice. J Exp Zool **196:**361, 1976.

10. Cunha GR, Lung B, Kato K: Role of the epithelial-stromal interaction during the development and expression of ovary-independent vaginal hyperplasia. Devel Biol **56:**52, 1977.

11. Fenoglio CM, Ferenczy A, Richart RM, et al: Scanning and transmission electron microscopic studies of vaginal adenosis and the cervical transformation zone in progeny exposed in utero to diethylstilbestrol. Amer J Obstet Gynecol **126:**170, 1976.

12. Forsberg JG: Late effects in the vaginal and cervical epithelia after injections of diethylstilbestrol into neonatal mice. Amer J Obstet Gynecol **121:**101, 1975.

13. Fu YS, Reagan JW, Hawliczek S, et al: The use of cellular studies in the investigation of the DES-exposed woman, in *Intrauterine Exposure to Diethylstilbestrol in the Human,* Herbst AL (ed.), Amer Coll Obstet Gynecol, 1978, pp. 34–44.

14. Hart WR, Townsend DE, Aldrich JO, et al: Histopathologic spectrum of vaginal adenosis and related changes in stilbestrol-exposed females. Cancer **37:**763, 1976.

15. Hart WR, Azharov I, Kaplan BJ, et al: Cytologic findings in stilbestrol exposed females with emphasis on detection of vaginal adenosis. Acta Cytol **20:**7, 1976.

16. Heinonen OP, Slone D, Monson RR, et al: Cardiovascular birth defects and antenatal exposure to female sex hormones. N Engl J Med **296:**267, 1977.

17. Henderson BE, Benton B, Cosgrove M, et al: Urogenital tract abnormalities in sons of women treated with diethylstilbestrol. Pediatrics **58:**505, 1976.

18. Herbst AL, Cole P, Colton T, et al: Age-incidence and risk of diethylstilbestrol-related clear cell adenocarcinoma of the vagina and cervix. Amer J Obstet Gynecol **128:**43, 1977.

19. Herbst AL, Poskanzer DC, Robboy SJ, et al: Prenatal exposure to stilbestrol. A prospective comparison of exposed female offspring with unexposed controls. N Engl J Med **292:**334, 1975.

20. Herbst AL, Robboy SJ, Scully RE, et al: Clear-cell adenocarcinoma of the vagina and cervix in girls: an analysis of 170 registry cases. Amer J Obstet Gynecol **119:**713, 1974.

21. Jones LA, Bern HA: Long-term effects of neonatal treatment with progesterone, alone and in combination with estrogen, on the mammary gland and reproductive tract of female BALB/cfC3H mice. Cancer Res **37**:67, 1977.

22. Jukes TH: Diethylstilbestrol in beef production: what is the risk to consumers? Prevent Med **5**:438, 1976.

23. Kaplan NM: Male pseudohermaphrodism. Report of a case with observations on pathogenesis. N Engl J Med **261**:641, 1959.

24. Kaufman RH, Binder GL, Gray PM, et al: Upper genital tract changes associated with exposure in utero to diethylstilbestrol. Amer J Obstet Gynecol **128**:51, 1977.

25. Kurman RJ, Scully RE: The incidence and histogenesis of vaginal adenosis: an autopsy study. Human Pathol **5**:265, 1974.

26. Labarth DR, Adam E, Noller KL, et al: Design and preliminary observations of national cooperative diethylstilbestrol adenosis (DESAD) project. Obstet Gynecol **51**:453, 1978.

27. Mattingly RF, Stafl A: Cancer risk in diethylstilbestrol-exposed offspring. Amer J Obstet Gynecol **126**:543, 1976.

28. McLachlan JA: Prenatal exposure to diethylstilbestrol in mice: toxicological studies. J Toxicol Environ Health **2**:527, 1977.

29. McLachlan JA, Newbold RR, Bullock B: Reproductive tract lesions in male mice exposed prenatally to diethylstilbestrol. Science **190**:991, 1975.

30. Miller RK, Heckmann ME, Reich KA: The pharmacokinetics of diethylstilbestrol in the pregnant rat. Gynecol Invest **8**:85, 1977 (Abst.).

31. Miller RK, Reich KA, Heckmann ME: Diethylstilbestrol: placental transfer, metabolism, and fetal distribution. Teratology **15**:20A, 1977 (Abst.).

32. Ng ABP, Reagan JW, Nadji M, et al: Natural history of vaginal adenosis in women exposed to diethylstilbestrol in utero. J Reprod Med **18**:1, 1977.

33. Pietras RJ, Szego CM, Mangan DE, et al: Elevated serum cathepsin B1 activity with vaginal adenosis and adenocarcinoma in young semen exposed in utero to diethylstilbestrol. Fed Proc **36**:387, 1977 (Abst.).

33a. Pixley E: Morphology of the fetal and prepubertal cervicovaginal epithelium, in *The Cervix*, Jordon JA, Singer A (eds.), Philadelphia, WB Saunders, 1976, p. 75.

34. Puri S, Fenoglio CM, Richart RM, et al: Clear cell carcinoma of cervix and vagina in progeny of women who received diethylstilbestrol: three cases with scanning and transmission electron microscopy. Amer J Obstet Gynecol **128**:550, 1977.

35. Robboy SJ, Friedlander LM, Welch WR, et al: Cytology of 575 young women with prenatal exposure to diethylstilbestrol. Obstet Gynecol **48**:511, 1976.

36. Robboy SJ, Herbst AL, Scully RE: Clear-cell adenocarcinoma of the genital tract in young females. Analysis of 37 tumors that persisted or recurred after primary therapy. Cancer **34**:606, 1974.

37. Robboy SJ, Keh PC, Nickerson RJ, et al: Squamous cell dysplasia and carcinoma in-situ after prenatal exposure to diethylstilbestrol: examination and follow-up of 1,424 females. Obstet Gynecol, May 1978.

38. Robboy SJ, Prat J, Welch WR, et al: Squamous cell neoplasia controversy in the DES-exposed female. Human Pathol **8**:483, 1977.

39. Robboy SJ, Scully RE, Herbst AL: Pathology of vaginal and cervical abnormalities associated with prenatal exposure to diethylstilbestrol (DES). J Reprod Med **15**:13, 1975.

40. Robboy SJ, Scully RE, Welch WR: Intrauterine diethylstilbestrol exposure and its consequences. Pathologic characteristics of vaginal adenosis, clear cell adenocarcinoma, and related lesions. Arch Pathol Lab Med **101**:1, 1977.

41. Robboy SJ, Welch WR: Microglandular hyperplasia in vaginal adenosis associated with oral contraceptives and prenatal diethylstilbestrol exposure. Obstet Gynecol **49**:430, 1977.

42. Sandberg EC: The incidence and distribution of occult vaginal adenosis. Amer J Obstet Gynecol **101**:322, 1968.

43. Sandberg EC: Benign cervical and vaginal changes associated with exposure to stilbestrol in utero. Amer J Obstet Gynecol **125**:777, 1976.

44. Schwartz RW, Stewart NB: Psychological effects of diethylstilbestrol exposure. J Amer Med Ass **237**:252, 1977.

45. Scully RE, Robboy SJ, Welch WR: Pathology and pathogenesis of diethylstilbestrol-related disorders of the female genital tract. In *Intrauterine Exposure to Diethylstilbestrol in the Human.* Herbst AL (ed.), Amer Coll Obstet Gynecol, 1978, pp. 8–22.

46. Shah HC, McLachlan JA: The fate of diethylstilbestrol in the pregnant mouse. J Pharmacol Exp Ther **197**:687, 1976.

47. Stafl A, Mattingly RF: Vaginal adenosis—a precancerous lesion? Amer J Obstet Gynecol **120**:666, 1974.

48. Taft PD, Robboy SJ, Herbst AL., et al: Cytology of clear-cell adenocarcinoma of the genital tract in young females. Report of 95 cases from registry. Acta Cytol **18**:279, 1974.

49. Ulfelder H, Robboy SJ: The embryologic development of the human vagina. Amer J Obstet Gynecol **126**:769, 1976.

50. Welch WR, Prat J, Robboy SJ, et al: Pathology of prenatal diethylstilbestrol (DES) exposure. Pathol Ann. In press.

51. Welch WR, Townsend DE, Robboy SJ, et al: Histologic findings following colposcopic examination of DES-exposed females. Key Biscayne, Fla., Society of Gynecological Oncology, January 1977 (Abst.).

52. Plapinger L, Unpublished results, 1978.

DISCUSSION

Question: What is the status on fertility in DES-exposed women?

Dr. Robboy: Current data indicate that the women we have followed are fertile. I hope within a year to be able to provide comparative rates for exposed and nonexposed women. A concern to many is whether deformities of the cervix that exposed women have may result in higher rates of abortion. Studies at the University of Chicago indicate that minor anatomic abnormalities of the genitourinary tract occur in males; severe sperm abnormalities have been found in many of these subjects. John McLachlan has reported that 60% of exposed male offspring of mice are infertile, having fibrotic testes located abnormally within the abdominal cavity.

Dr. Gerald Cunha: Your study points out the possible long-term effects incurred by exposure of developing organisms to very potent steroid and nonsteroid sex hormones. Unfortunately, in the past, communication between the experimental biologist and clinician has been rather poor. Diethylstilbestrol is probably the best example of this point. As early as the 1960s, experimental biologists showed that exposure to estrogens during early critical periods of development resulted in severe lesions. Unfortunately, these data were not widely publicized, and DES was administered for an additional 10 or more years. Today, as a result of a study published in 1976 in *The New England Journal of Medicine* by Johnson et al., 17-hydroxyprogesterone caproate is now being used in humans to extend the gestational period. Another study, by Lovell Jones, which is now only in abstract form but will be published soon by the University of California, has demonstrated that in mice exposure to progesterone leads to vaginal cancer in a very high incidence later in life.

Dr. Robboy: I have reviewed the slides prepared by Dr. Jones. Although the tumor is not similar morphologically to the clear-cell adenocarcinoma that develops in humans, I agree with your thesis that exposure to hormones during embryogenesis may lead in the future to other cancers that are not yet known or recognized.

Dr. Morris: Forsberg has shown that estradiol as well as other estrogens produces exactly the same amount of adenosis as DES. I suspect that any estrogen will have the same effect, but DES just happened to be the estrogen clinicians used. Also, there has been no demonstration in animals that administration of the hormone to the mother induces cancer in the fetus. In the neonatal mice studies, the estrogen is given after the mouse is born, which is different from administration to the mother. In our own work in rhesus monkeys, we have not been able to demonstrate adenosis. Our results, however, reflect an inadequate number of experiments and inadequate time and duration of administration.

Dr. Robboy: We began studying monkeys about three years ago, but unfortunately there is a long interval between the time of initial injection and the time the offspring are postpubertal. I agree with you that there is no report of an animal model in which transplacental exposure to the fetus has resulted in development of a cancer. Another point this brings up is that we should be careful not to say that DES is definitely a transplacental carcinogen. The drug certainly passes through the placenta, but it may be that it functions as a teratogen, resulting in congenital anomalies. These anomalies, after secondary exposure to some other environmental factor or endogenous hormone, may eventually result in cancer.

Dr. Morris: We are limited by the supposition that one in 1000 monkeys will develop adenocarcinoma. A monkey costs about $1,000 a year to maintain. To carry out that experiment you would have to buy 2000 baby monkeys, because half will be male. At the end of 15 years, if any one of us tried to report in a medical journal the development of only one adenocarcinoma, I do not believe that DES would be accepted as etiologic.

Dr. Silverberg: Dr. Morris' point is well taken. We should have emphasized it earlier. I agree that there is probably not much difference between one estrogen and another, and I think that those of you who are clinicians are now being bombarded by messages that "our estrogen is better than their estrogen" because there is less risk involved. I think that any estrogen that is administered will be metabolized eventually to the same end product. If one estrogen is harmful, they probably all are. Someone raised the question of whether adenosis is a premalignant lesion. Would you comment about this, Dr. Robboy?

Dr. Robboy: I believe that adenosis is a benign condition, but that it gives rise to an atypical (i.e., dysplastic) form of adenosis, which may have a premalignant potential, albeit small.

Question: How may patients with known adenosis have developed adenocarcinoma? How do you follow women with adenosis without carcinoma, and what should you tell them to do?

Dr. Robboy: I tell them not to worry and to come back next year for another examination. Not one of the 1500 women we have followed has developed a carcinoma during the follow-up period.

Question: Why should women with mild adenosis or a hood not take oral contraceptives?

Dr. Robboy: I have no specific data to suggest that use of oral contraceptives in DES-exposed females is contraindicated. I do feel, though, that any patient willing to use this form of medication must recognize that complications may occur, such as the recently reported hepatomas. On the other hand, the complications of a therapeutic abortion are probably much worse than the theoretical and already known complications of oral contraceptives.

Progesterone and Estrogen Receptors in Cancer Treatment

Clarence E. Ehrlich, M.D.
Peter C. M. Young, Ph.D.
Lawrence H. Einhorn, M.D.

Manipulations of the steroid hormone milieu have become accepted modalities of therapy in breast cancer (1), endometrial cancer (2), leukemia and lymphomatous disease (3), and prostatic cancer (4). While objective responses occur in a significant number of these tumors, many fail to respond. The patients whose tumors fail to respond are subjected to ineffective therapy for a period of time, during which their tumors grow. Since additive or ablative hormonal therapy may entail risk to the patient, especially since alternate therapies are available for each of these tumors, a method of selecting hormonally responsive tumors could improve their management.

While Beatson (5, 6) observed regression of breast cancer in two patients after castration nearly 80 years ago, the first indication that breast cancer cells contained a specific mechanism for interaction with steroid hormones was provided by Folca et al. in 1961 (7). These investigators observed that after injection of labeled hexestrol into women with breast cancer, the tumors of patients with breast cancer who responded favorably to adrenalectomy incorporated more radioactivity than did those that did not respond.

Jensen et al. (8) and Gorski et al. (9) in 1968 independently suggested a "two-step mechanism" for the association of 17β-estradiol with target cells. The proposed two-step mechanism that occurs after interaction of a steroid hormone with a target cell can be described as follows:

1. The steroid enters the cell by diffusion through the plasma membrane, binds to a specific steroid receptor protein in the cytoplasm, which is then activated by a temperature- and salt-dependent process, forming a so-called transformed steroid-receptor complex.
2. The activated complex is then translocated, possibly by simple diffusion to the

nucleus, where nuclear receptor complex binds to acceptor protein(s) on the chromatin.

3. This translocation of the steroid-receptor complex to the nucleus, along with its binding to chromatin, facilitates the synthesis of different RNAs by activating RNA polymerases and increasing chromatin template activity.

Subsequent studies in vitro and in vivo from several laboratories have confirmed this mechanism of action for steroid hormones (10–12). Because of the crucial role of cytoplasmic receptors in steroid hormone action in normal target tissue, investigations were undertaken to study both the qualitative and quantitative aspects of the receptors in known or suspected steroid-responsive tumors with the hope that some parameters could be found that would be predictive a priori of a response to steroid hormone manipulation. The role of receptors in cancer treatment will be reviewed in breast cancer and endometrial adenocarcinoma primarily because this topic has been our main interest, clinically and in terms of research goals.

BREAST CANCER

Because the breast is the target organ of a wide variety of steroid and protein hormones, it is not surprising that endocrine factors play a role in the induction and subsequent proliferation of breast neoplasms. As early as 1836, Cooper (13) observed a correlation between tumor growth and the menstrual cycle, and later in the same century, Beatson (5) reported the regression of metastatic lesions after oophorectomy in premenopausal women with advanced breast cancer. In 1952, Huggins and Bergenstal (14) reported remission of advanced breast cancer in postmenopausal women after bilateral adrenalectomy. Luft et al. (15) and Pearson and Ray (16) observed similar remissions after hypophysectomy. Attempts to select hormonally responsive breast cancers through the use of urinary steroid excretion rates (21, 22) or in vivo uptake of labeled estrogen derivatives by breast cancers (7, 23) have been ineffective or impractical.

ESTROGEN RECEPTORS IN BREAST CANCER

In 1971, Jensen et al. (17) reported a correlation between the amount of cytoplasmic estrogen receptors (ER) in breast cancers and their response to endocrine ablation or hormone administration. Their results were confirmed by others from several laboratories (18–20).

In 1974, a workshop held under the auspices of the Breast Cancer Task Force of the National Cancer Institute determined that there is a correlation between the presence of ER and the response to hormone manipulation in breast cancer (1). In addition, evidence was presented that indicates that:

1. Tumors from postmenopausal patients contained higher ER values than did those from premenopausal patients.

2. No correlation was found between the histologic type of tumor and the presence of ER.

3. There was a negative correlation between the size of the primary tumor and the presence of ER.

4. There was no correlation between the clinical stage of the patient and tumor ER.

5. There was no correlation between positive or negative axillary lymph nodes and the presence of ER in the primary tumor.

6. About 60% of primary tumors were reported to contain ER.

7. There was no correlation with the location of the tumor in the breast and the presence of ER.

8. There was no correlation between disease-free interval and ER or between absolute ER value and duration of remission.

9. There does not appear to be a linear relationship between the absolute value for tumor ER and the percentage of patients who respond to endocrine therapy.

10. The ability of ER values in predicting a response to endocrine therapy is equal for primary and metastatic tumors.

11. Data from this study correlating ER and endocrine responsiveness can be summarized as follows:
    a. Ablative therapy. Of 127 patients with negative tumor ER values, only 5% responded, while 58% of patients with positive tumor ER values responded.
    b. Additive therapy. Of 94 patients with negative tumor ER values, only 8% responded, whereas 60% of patients with positive tumor ER values responded.

Clinical observations indicate that only about 60% of patients' tumors that contain appreciable cytoplasmic ER respond to endocrine therapy (1). The question arises as to why the remaining 40% of ER-positive breast cancers are resistant to hormone manipulation. In the unresponsive ER-positive tumors, several explanations have been advanced to explain the clinical unresponsiveness (24, 25). First, the criteria for "positive" and "negative" may be inaccurate. In fact, Jensen et al. (26) recently redefined their criteria for positive and negative and now classify 70% of breast cancers as ER poor or low and 30% as ER rich. Second, tumors may not have homogeneous receptor populations. Enough cells with high concentrations of ER may be present in the biopsy specimen to give a positive assay, but too many ER poor cells may be present in the remaining tumor to prevent a clinical response. Third, the surgical ablative procedure may not remove sufficient endocrinologically active tissue. Several tissues, such as liver, fat, and skin, are capable of metabolizing estrogen precursors to biologically active estrone or estradiol (27). Fourth, the tumor may have active steroid-metabolizing enzymes that inactivate the administered hormone (28). Fifth, the defects may be distal to the initial steroid receptor interaction. Finally, the tumor may be dependent on other hormones, such as prolactin, growth hormone, or androgens.

PROGESTERONE RECEPTORS IN BREAST CANCER

Since only about 60% of patient's tumors with positive ER respond to endocrine therapy, attempts have been made to find additional markers of hormone-responsive tumors. It is known that in estrogen target tissues, the synthesis of progesterone receptors (PgR) is influenced by estrogen. Therefore, it is possible that the PgR might be a better marker of a hormone-responsive tumor, because a product of hormone action would appear to be a better parameter to use than would binding of the hormone to its receptor in assessing hormone dependency of a tumor (24). Subsequent evaluation of clinical response related to concentration of ER and PgR in breast cancer has revealed a 40% response rate in ER-positive/PgR-negative breast cancer in 15 patients. In 12 patients whose tumors were ER-positive/PgR-positive, 92% responded to hormone therapy.

We have determined ER and PgR in 138 breast cancers and have data on 29 cases involving a biopsy and response to a trial of endocrine therapy. The distributions of receptor combinations are shown in Table 1. We found that 53% of all breast cancers studied were ER positive, but only 38% of all tumors were positive for both PgR and ER. This percentage of PgR- and ER-positive tumors is close to the response rate of breast cancer to hormone therapy as reported by other groups of investigators (1). McGuire et al. (29) observed that PgR was rarely found in ER-negative breast cancers but was present in 59% of ER-positive tumors. Our preliminary data (Table 1) show that 26% of ER-negative tumors had detectable PgR, while 73% of ER-positive tumors were also PgR positive.

The data in Table 2 suggest that tumors that are ER- and PgR-positive have a greater likelihood of responding to hormone therapy. The response rate of 72%

Table 1. Distribution of Estrogen and Progesterone Receptors in 138 Breast Cancers

ER^{+a}	ER^-	ER^+, PgR^{+b}	ER^+, PgR^-	ER^-, PgR^+	ER^-, PgR^-
73/138	65/138	53/138	20/138	17/138	48/138
(53%)	(47%)	(38%)	(15%)	(12%)	(35%)

[a] Above 12 fmoles per milligram of cytosol protein.

[b] Above 6 fmoles per milligram of cytosol protein.

Table 2. Receptor Distribution and Response to Endocrine Therapy in 29 Breast Cancers

Receptor Distribution	Number of Responders	Response Rate (%)
$ER^{+,a} PgR^{+b}$	13/18	72
ER^+, PgR^-	1/7	14
ER^-, PgR^+	1/1	—
ER^-, PgR^-	1/3	—

[a] Above 12 fmoles per milligram of cytosol protein.

[b] Above 6 fmoles per milligram of cytosol protein.

for breast cancers that contain both ER and PgR appears to be considerably higher than that for tumors that lack either ER or PgR or both. Our results agree with those obtained by Horwitz and McGuire (81) in a slightly larger series of patients.

PROLACTIN AND GLUCOCORTICOID RECEPTORS IN BREAST CANCER

The role of prolactin in breast cancer is much less clear in man than in rodents (30). Limited evidence is available, which indicates that some human breast tumors may be dependent on prolactin for continued growth or maintaining their viability (31, 32). Prolactin receptors have been demonstrated in mouse, rat, and rabbit mammary tissue and tumors (33–37), and the concentrations of receptor sites seemed to correlate with the responsiveness of the tumors to prolactin (34, 35). Although very little is known about prolactin receptors in normal or carcinomatous human mammary cells, one would be inclined to think that a similar receptor-response relationship could exist in human breast tissue. Unfortunately, reduction of prolactin levels with bromoergocryptine, an inhibitor of prolactin secretion, has not proved to be of value in the treatment of metastatic breast cancer (38). It is possible that a more potent inhibitor is required for successful treatment, because it has been shown that there is correlation between near-zero serum prolactin concentrations and breast tumor regression in some patients after hypophysectomy (32). At any rate, the effect of low serum prolactin levels on growth of breast tumors needs to be reevaluated, particularly in those tumors demonstrated to be prolactin dependent in vitro. Studies on prolactin receptor in human breast cancer may provide just the tool for this purpose.

Androgens and corticosteroids have also been used for treatment of advanced breast cancers. Objective regression was observed in about 20% of the tumors treated with androgens (39). The use of corticosteroids gave even less satisfactory results (40), but such treatment may have value in tumors metastatic to certain sites, such as the lung and brain. The site(s) of action of these steroid hormones in breast cancer is not clear. It is believed that corticosteroids probably produce their effects partially by suppression of adrenal function. Glucocorticoid receptor has been demonstrated in normal mouse mammary gland (41), mouse mammary tumor (42, 43), and in human mammary carcinoma (82). Evidence for the presence of androgen receptor in human breast tumor has also been documented (83). Although it has been suggested that androgen receptor could serve as a marker of hormone-responsive breast tumors (84), sufficient data are not available for evaluation of its clinical significance. It is, therefore, of interest to also study glucocorticoid and androgen receptors in human breast cancer and to correlate the receptor contents with clinical response of these tumors to hormonal manipulation.

ENDOMETRIAL CANCER

In 1960, Kelley and Baker described objective tumor response of metastatic endometrial adenocarcinoma in seven of 22 patients treated with a progestin

(46). Subsequent clinical experience has shown an objective regression or arrest of tumor growth for various periods of time in about one third of patients treated with progesterone or progestins (47–50). The factor(s) that predisposes endometrial adenocarcinomas to respond to progestational agents has eluded investigators. Anderson (51) proposed that progesterone acts on endometrial adenocarcinoma through immunologic mechanisms, by altering endogenous hormone status, or through a direct cellular effect. No evidence is available to support the first two hypotheses, but results obtained from several studies suggest a direct cellular effect (52, 53).

In studies with explanted cultures, Nordqvist found that culture of one endometrial adenocarcinoma was inhibited by norhydroxyprogesterone, while another histologically identical carcinoma was not affected (53). The effect of steroid hormones on endometrial carcinoma in organ cultures is also variable. Low concentrations of both 17β-estradiol and progesterone were found to have a marginal effect on tissue survival, whereas a high dose of progesterone markedly reduces the survival of the tumor tissue (54–57). Such a dose usually causes necrosis and may well represent a general toxic effect on the cells.

Progestational agents injected into the uterine cavity of patients with previously untreated endometrial carcinoma cause severe degeneration of the cancer cells (58, 59), similar to that observed in organ cultures. It is interesting to note that progesterone lowers the uptake of oxygen in vitro (60) and reduces the synthesis of DNA and RNA in normal (61) and carcinomatous human endometria (7) in short-term incubations in vitro. Since carcinomas of the bowel and stomach do not show any response to progesterone in vitro (57), the possibility of a nonspecific effect of the hormone seems unlikely. Attempts to correlate the degree of response with tumor grade and patient's age have failed.

PROGESTERONE RECEPTORS IN ENDOMETRIAL CANCER

The primary treatment for recurrent or advanced endometrial adenocarcinoma is with progestins, even though only one of three endometrial adenocarcinomas respond. Therefore, the majority of patients with advanced or recurrent endometrial adenocarcinoma thus treated are subjected to a trial of ineffective therapy. Selection of therapy based on clinical characteristics of the patient or tumor alone has failed to improve treatment results (62). A laboratory test that could accurately predict a priori progesterone sensitivity of the tumor would prevent delay in initiating appropriate treatment and would help the physician select the proper therapy in a rational way.

Assuming that progesterone and estrogen act on human endometrium and mammary gland through similar mechanisms, one would anticipate that measurement of PgR and/or ER in endometrial adenocarcinoma could identify tumors that are likely to respond and define those in which response is less probable. We hypothesized that cytoplasmic PgR rather than ER would be the most likely predictor of response for two reasons: progestins are used to treat recurrent or advanced endometrial adenocarcinoma, and the production of cytoplasmic PgR is an end-product of estrogen action, and thus its presence indicates a functioning ER system (81).

Specific cytoplasmic PgR that bind [^{3}H]progesterone in vitro have been demonstrated and characterized in normal, hyperplastic, and carcinomatous human endometria (63–69). To evaluate the relationship between cytoplasmic PgR and response of endometrial adenocarcinomas to progestins, a study was initiated at the Department of Obstetrics and Gynecology of Indiana University Medical Center in 1974. We have studied progesterone binding in endometria and various gynecologic tumors from 149 patients by use of a simple dextran-coated charcoal assay. The tissue samples included normal endometria, endometrial polyps, endometrial cystic and adenomatous hyperplasia, adenocarcinoma of the endometrium, and a variety of gynecologic tumors.

The breaking point between high and low PgR was arbitrarily chosen to be 50 femtomoles (fmol) per milligram of cytosol protein, since the highest PgR observed in nonendometrial gynecologic cancers and other miscellaneous tissue was 49 fmol per milligram of cytosol protein.

From Table 3, it is apparent that all normal endometria, except one, had high PgR levels. The mean PgR value for proliferative endometria (587.9 fmol/mg of cytosol protein) is greater than the mean PgR for secretory endometria (327.7 fmol/mg of cytosol protein). These results are in agreement with the findings of others (65, 66, 70).

Five of six endometrial polyps and 15 of 18 endometrial hyperplasias had high PgR levels. The proliferative endometria and endometrial hyperplasias had similar mean PgR concentrations (Table 3). No association is seen between type of hyperplasia and amount of PgR. There were four cystic, six cystic and adenomatous, and eight adenomatous hyperplasias. One cystic and two mixed cystic and adenomatous hyperplasias had low PgR values. All pure adenomatous hyperplasias had high PgR levels.

Since it has been shown that production of PgR is dependent on estrogen stimulation of the target cells (71, 72), and because both proliferative and hyperplastic endometria result from estrogen stimulation, it is not surprising that these endometria should have the highest PgR concentrations.

Several laboratories have shown that certain endometrial adenocarcinomas retain specific cytoplasmic PgR in appreciable concentrations (66, 67, 70, 71). In our study, the PgR of 53 nonirradiated endometrial adenocarcinomas were measured. These data show a progressive loss of PgR from the well-differentiated (grade I) to the anaplastic (grade III) endometrial adenocar-

Table 3. Progesterone Binding by Normal and Hyperplastic Endometria

Tissue Examined	Number of Patients	Endometria with High PgR Activity[a] (%)
Normal endometria		
Proliferative	15	100
Secretory	16	94
Endometrial hyperplasia	18	83
Endometrial polyps	6	83

[a] Above 50 fmoles per milligram of cytosol protein.

Table 4. Progesterone Binding by Endometrial Adenocarcinomas and Sarcomas

Grade of Tumor	Number of Patients	Tumors with High PgR Activity[a] (%)
I	19	84
II	17	47
IV	17	24
Irradiated tumors	10	10
Endometrial sarcomas		
Stromal	6	33
Mixed mullerian	4	25
Miscellaneous gynecologic	11	0

[a] Above 50 fmoles per milligram of cytosol protein.

cinomas (Table 4). If PgR play a role in a tumor's response to progestin therapy, these data could explain why the response rate is higher in well-differentiated endometrial adenocarcinomas than in anaplastic tumors (50).

We have examined 10 endometrial adenocarcinomas from within irradiated fields and found that nine of 10 had low PgR values (Table 4). Some of these tumors were assayed immediately after irradiation and others years after irradiation. The lack of cytoplasmic PgR in irradiated tumors is consistent with the clinical observation that response to progestin is decreased in irradiated patients (50).

We have examined 10 endometrial sarcomas for the presence of cytoplasmic PgR. Again using a value of 50 fmol per milligram of cytosol protein as the criterion, two of six (33%) stromal sarcomas and one of four (25%) mixed mullerian sarcomas were found to have high PgR levels (Table 4).

In an attempt to evaluate the role of PgR in the response of endometrial adenocarcinomas to progestin therapy, 16 endometrial adenocarcinomas were assayed for the presence of PgR prior to initiating therapy with medroxyprogesterone acetate. The results of these studies are shown in Table 5. All five tumors with high PgR values showed an objective response, whereas only one of 11 tumors with low PgR activity responded. Two endometrial stromal sarcomas

Table 5. Relationship Between Response of Endometrial Adenocarcinomas to Progestin and Progesterone Receptor Levels

PgR Activity	Responders		Nonresponders
	Partial	Complete	
High	5	0	0
Low	0	1	12[a]

[a] Includes two endometrial stromal sarcomas.

with low PgR levels were treated with medroxyprogesterone acetate, and both failed to respond. High concentrations of PgR appear to correlate with a response to progestin therapy and low PgR with a lack of response to progestin therapy. These data strongly suggest that PgR may be used to select therapy for recurrent or advanced endometrial adenocarcinomas much as ER is used to determine therapy for advanced breast cancer (1). Such an approach is outlined in Figure 1.

The approach outlined in Figure 1 would allow patients with high PgR levels who would benefit from progestin therapy to receive appropriate therapy and patients with low PgR to be started on cytotoxic chemotherapy. Patients in the low-PgR group would benefit, in that they would be started on appropriate therapy earlier and thus avoid 2–3 months of ineffective therapy. Since it is a well-accepted principle of chemotherapy that the smaller the tumor volume, the better the chance for response, these PgR-negative tumors would potentially have a better chance to respond to cytotoxic chemotherapy. According to the available data in the literature, response rates to cytotoxic chemotherapy of endometrial adenocarcinomas range from 25 to 28%. If this response rate, or possibly a better response rate, could be added to that obtained with progestin treatment, a substantial improvement in therapy of advanced or recurrent endometrial adenocarcinoma would be anticipated.

The role of adjuvant progestins in primary treatment of endometrial adenocarcinomas remains controversial (51, 74, 75). We think that since recur-

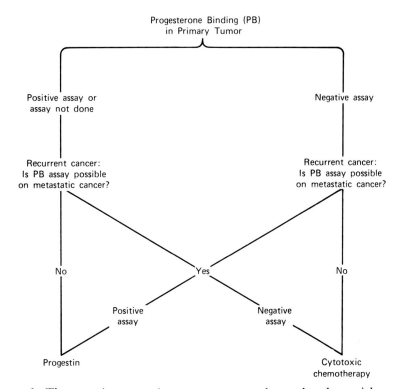

Figure 1. Therapeutic approach to recurrent or advanced endometrial cancer.

rence and failure are greatest in patients with stages I_{G2}, I_{G3}, II, III, and deep myometrial invasion, patients in these stages whose tumors have high PgR values might benefit from adjuvant progestin therapy. However, this hypothesis remains to be confirmed. Since we could not detect any PgR activity in most irradiated tumors, progestins are of questionable value for treating tumor within the radiation field.

ESTROGEN RECEPTORS IN ENDOMETRIAL CANCER

The usefulness of ER in predicting a response of advanced or recurrent endometrial adenocarcinoma to progestin therapy is uncertain. Specific cytoplasmic ER has been demonstrated in normal and abnormal endometria (67, 69, 76–78). While Evans et al. (77) and Terenius et al. (78) found that the ER concentration correlated with the degree of differentiation of the tumor (welldifferentiated tumors showing a higher concentration than poorly differentiated tumors), Pollow et al. (67) noted that the concentrations of binding sites for 17-β estradiol were low in endometrial carcinomas that were well differentiated and high in undifferentiated tumors.

More recently, Kontula et al. (69) reported that both ER and PgR were present in 26 of 32 endometrial adenocarcinomas studied. Only ER activity was detected in four tumors, while two others did not contain either receptor. It was also observed that the well-differentiated adenocarcinomas seemed to contain higher ER and PgR activities than did the poorly differentiated cancers. These authors noted that the PgR/ER ratio was clearly higher in nonmalignant (PgR/ER ratio ranged from 4 to 6) than in malignant (PgR/ER ratio ranged from 0.5 to 2) endometrial tissue (69). Our results on the distribution of ER and PgR in 22 endometrial cancers evaluated in our laboratory are presented in Table 6. It

Table 6. Progesterone and Estrogen Receptor Distributions in Endometrial Adenocarcinomas

Receptor Distribution	Grade I	Grade II	Grade III	Total
PgR+,[a] ER+[b]	4/7 (57%)	5/11 (45%)	0/4 —	9/22 (41%)
PgR+, ER−	2/7 (29%)	1/11 (9%)	1/4 (25%)	4/22 (18%)
PgR−, ER+	0/7 —	1/11 (9%)	0/4 —	1/22 (5%)
PgR−, ER−	1/7 (14%)	4/11 (36%)	3/4 (75%)	8/22 (36%)

[a] Above 50 fmoles per milligram of cytosol protein.

[b] Above 12 fmoles per milligram of cytosol protein.

appeared that more of the well-differentiated tumors tend to have higher concentrations of both ER and PgR; with increasing tumor anaplasia, more of these tumors lost both ER and PgR. The role of ER in the treatment of endometrial adenocarcinomas remains to be shown.

EPITHELIAL OVARIAN CANCER

There are few published clinical trials of high-dose progestin or estrogen therapy for ovarian cancer. The reported response rates to progestin therapy vary from 9 to 65% (79). In a recent review article, Tobias and Griffiths (79) reported that a cumulative response rate of 38% was observed in 60 ovarian cancers treated with progestins. There is one report in the literature of ovarian cancer treatment with estrogens, in which two responses were reported in 14 patients (80).

We have studied 19 ovarian epithelial cancers for the presence of PgR and ER (Table 7). It is apparent that some of these tumors contain specific cytoplasmic

Table 7. Progesterone and Estrogen Receptor Distributions in 19 Epithelial Cancers of the Ovary

Receptor Status	Primary Ovarian Cancer	Metastasis
PgR$^+$,^{a} ER^{+b}	10/19 (53%)	2/4
PgR$^+$, ER$^-$	2/19 (11%)	1/4
PgR$^-$, ER$^+$	4/19 (21%)	0
PgR$^-$, ER$^-$	3/19 (15%)	1/4

^{a} Above 6 fmoles per milligram of cytosol protein.

^{b} Above 12 fmoles per milligram of cytosol protein.

steroid receptors for progesterone and estrogen. The clinical significance of these observations is unknown, but their presence might be predictive of a clinical response by these tumors to hormonal therapy. Further studies are planned in this area.

SUMMARY

Cancers that arise from target tissues of steroid hormones frequently remain responsive to these hormones. Responses to endocrine manipulation by breast cancer, endometrial cancer, leukemia, lymphomatous diseases, and prostatic cancer are well documented, but a significant number of these cancers fail to respond to hormone therapy.

The increase in our understanding of the mechanism of action of steroid hormones, the recognition of the crucial role played by specific cytoplasmic steroid receptors in this mechanism, and the development of methods for measurement of cytoplasmic steroid receptors have allowed physicians to formulate a more rational and effective approach to endocrine therapy of hormonally responsive cancers. The use of ER and PgR as markers of hormonally responsive tumors has improved the response rate in breast cancers treated with hormonal manipulation. Patients whose tumors contain both PgR and ER appear to have a much higher response rate than do those that lack one or the other receptor or both.

Specific cytoplasmic PgR have been found in normal and carcinomatous endometria. As in the breast cancers, the presence of these receptors in endometrial cancers seems to be associated with a response of the tumors to hormone (progestin) therapy, while their absence appears to indicate otherwise.

Epithelial cancers of the ovary have been reported to respond to hormonal manipulation. Recent studies have demonstrated the presence of specific cytoplasmic ER and PgR in these cancers. Whether these receptors could also be used as markers of hormonally responsive ovarian tumors remains to be shown.

REFERENCES

1. McGuire WL, Carbone PP, Vollmar EP: *Estrogen Receptors in Human Breast Cancer*, New York, Raven Press, 1975, p. 1.
2. Reifenstein EC: Gynecol Oncol **2**:377, 1974.
3. Lippman ME, Halterman RH, Leventhal BG, et al: J Clin Invest **52**:1715, 1973.
4. Huggins C: J Amer Med Ass **131**:576, 1946.
5. Beatson GT: Lancet **ii**:104, 1896.
6. Hayward J: *Hormones and Breast Cancer*, London, Heinemann, 1970.
7. Folca PJ, Glaslock RF, and Jruin WT: Lancet **2**:796, 1961.
8. Jensen EV, Suzuki T, Kawashima T, et al: Proc Nat Acad Sci USA **59**:632, 1968.
9. Gorski J, Toff DO, Shyamala G, et al: Recent Progr Hormone Res **24**:45, 1968.
10. Jensen EV, DeSombre ER: Annu Rev Biochem **41**:203, 1972.
11. O'Malley BW, Means AR: Science **183**:510, 1974.
12. King RJB, Mainwaring WIP: *Steroid Cell Interactions*, Baltimore, University Park Press, 1974.
13. Cooper AP: *The Principles and Practice of Surgery*, London, E. Cop, 1836, vol. 1.
14. Huggins C, Bergenstal DM: Cancer Res **12**:134, 1952.
15. Luft R, Olivecrona H, Ikkos D, et al: in *Endocrine Aspects of Breast Cancer*, Currie AR (ed.), Edinburgh, Livingstone, 1958, p. 27.
16. Pearson OH, Ray BS: Amer J Surg **99**:544, 1960.
17. Jensen EV, Block GE, Smith S, et al: Nat Cancer Inst Monogr **34**:55, 1971.
18. Maass H, Engel B, Holmeister H, et al: Amer J Obstet Gynecol **113**:377, 1972.
19. Engelsman E, Persijn JP, Korsten CB, et al: Brit Med J **2**:750, 1973.
20. Leung BS, Fletcher WS, Lindell TD, et al: Arch Surg **106**:515, 1973.
21. Bulbrook RD, Greenwood FC, Hayward JL: Lancet **1**:1154, 1960.
22. Bulbrook RD, Hayward JL: Cancer Res **25**:1135, 1965.
23. Braunsberg H, James VHT, Irvine WT, et al: Lancet **1**:163, 1973.
24. Horwitz KB, McGuire WL, Pearson OH, et al: Science **189**:726, 1975.
25. Lippman M: Life Sci **18**:143, 1976.
26. Jensen EV, Smith S, DeSombre ER: J Steroid Biochem **7**:911, 1976.
27. Siiteri PK, Williams JE, Takaki NK: J Steroid Biochem **7**:897, 1976.
28. Adams JB, Wong MSF: J Endocrinol **44**:69, 1969.
29. McGuire WL, Horwitz KB, Pearson OH, et al: Cancer **39**:2934, 1977.
30. McGuire WL, Chamness GC, Costlow ME, et al: Metabolism **23**:75, 1974.
31. Salih H, Flax H, Brander W, et al: Lancet **2**:1103, 1972.
32. Hobbs JR, Salih H, Flax H, et al: Proc Roy Soc Med **66**:866, 1973.
33. Costlow ME, Buschow RA, McGuire WL: Science **184**:85, 1974.

34. Turkington RW: Cancer Res **34:**758, 1974.
35. Guerzon P, Pensky J, Pearson OH: Program of the 56th Annual Meeting of the Endocrine Society, June 1974, p. 244.
36. Frantz WL, MacIndoe JH, Turkington RW: J Endocrinol **60:**485, 1974.
37. Shiu RPC, Friesen HG: Biochem J **140:**301, 1974.
38. European Breast Cancer Group: Eur J Cancer **8:**155, 1972.
39. Goldenberg IS, Sedransk N, Volk H, et al: Cancer **36:**308, 1975.
40. Van Gilse NA: Cancer Chemother Rep **16:**293, 1962.
41. Shyamala G: Biochemistry **12:**3085, 1973.
42. Shyamala G: J Biol Chem **249:**2160, 1974.
43. Shyamala G: Biochemistry **14:**437, 1975.
44. Engelsman E, Korsten CB, Persijn JP, et al: Brit J Cancer **30:**177, 1974.
45. Raith L, Wirtz A, Karl HJ: Klin Wochschr **52:**299, 1974.
46. Kelley RM, Baker WH: Nat Cancer Inst Monogr **9:**235, 1960.
47. Anderson DG: Amer J Obstet Gynecol **92:**87, 1965.
48. Kelley RM, Baker WH: Cancer Res **25:**1190, 1965.
49. Kistner RW, Griffiths CT, Craig JM: Cancer **18:**1563, 1965.
50. Smith JP: in *Cancer of the Uterus and Ovary*, Chicago, Yearbook Medical Publishers, 1969, p. 73.
51. Anderson DG: Amer J Obstet Gynecol **113:**195, 1972.
52. Nordqvist S: J Endocrinol **48:**29, 1970.
53. Nordqvist S: Acta Obstet Gynaecol Scand Suppl **19:**25, 1972.
54. Nordqvist S: Acta Obstet Gynaecol Scand **43:**296, 1964.
55. Kohorn EI, Tchao RJ: Obstet Gynaecol Brit Common **75:**1262, 1968.
56. Nordqvist S: Acta Obstet Gynaecol Scand **48**(Suppl 3):118, 1969.
57. Nordqvist S: Acta Obstet Gynaecol Scand **49:**275, 1970.
58. Truskett ID: in Symposium on Recent Advances in Ovarian and Synthetic Steroids, Sydney, Australia, 1964.
59. Kistner RW: Ob/Gyn Digest **17:**26, 1975.
60. Hackl H: Arch Gynaekol **203:**464, 1966.
61. Nordqvist RSB: J Endocrinol **48:**17, 1970.
62. Kohorn EI: Gynecol Oncol **4:**398, 1976.
63. Young PCM, Cleary RE: J Clin Endocrinol Metab **39:**425, 1974.
64. Young PCM, Ehrlich CE, Cleary RE: Amer J Obstet Gynecol **125:**353, 1976.
65. McLaughlin DT, Richardson GS: J Clin Endocrinol Metab **42:**667, 1976.
66. Haukkamaa M, Karjalainen O, Luukkainen T: Amer J Obstet Gynecol **111:**205, 1971.
67. Pollow K, Lubbert H, Boquoi E, et al: Endocrinology **96:**319, 1975.
68. Crocker SG, Milton PJD, Taylor RW, et al: in *Gynecologic Malignancy*, Brush MG, Taylor RW (eds.), Baltimore, Williams and Williams, 1975, p. 179.
69. Kontula K, Janne O, Kuppila A, et al: Abstract 2nd International Meeting on Endometrial Cancer and Related Subjects, St. Thomas Hospital, London, March 30–31, 1977.
70. Rao BR, Wiest WG, Allen WN: Endocrinology **95:**1275, 1974.
71. O'Malley BW, Sherman MR, Toft DO: Proc Nat Acad Sci USA **67:**501, 1970.
72. Milgrom E, Thi L, Atger M, et al: J Biol Chem **248:**6366, 1973.
73. Donovan JF: Cancer **34:**1587, 1974.
74. Lewis GC, Slack NH, Mortel R, et al: Gynecol Oncol **2:**368, 1974.
75. Boute J, Decoster JM, Ide P: Cancer **25:**907, 1970.
76. Crocker SG, Milton PJD, King RJB: J Endocrinol **62:**145, 1974.
77. Evans LH, Martin JD, Hahnel R: J Clin Endocrinol Metab **38:**23, 1974.

78. Terenius L, Lindell A, Persson BH: Cancer Res **31:**1895, 1971.

79. Tobias JS, Griffiths TC: N Engl J Med **294:**818, 1976.

80. Long RTL, Evans AM: Mod Med **60:**1125, 1963.

81. Horwitz KB, McGuire WL: in *Progesterone Receptors in Normal and Neoplastic Tissues*, McGuire WL, Raynaud JP, Baulieu EE (eds.), New York, Raven Press, 1977.

82. Fazeka AG, MacFarlane JK: Cancer Res **37:**640, 1977.

83. Wagner RK, Gorlich L, Jungblut PW: Acta Endocrinol Suppl **173:**65, 1973.

84. Engelsman E: in *Proceedings of the First E.O.R.T.C. Breast Cancer Working Conference*, Brussels, 1975, *Breast Cancer: Trends in Research and Treatment*, JC Heason, WM Mattheiem, and M Rozencweig (eds.), New York, Raven Press, 1976.

Index